ABBAS

SWORD
AND
SEIZURE

Muhammad's Epilepsy & Creation of Islam

To: Brode   MAR 1 '07

Brooks: Last Typing
Office Lumita
ABBAS

Sword and Seizure

Muhammad's Epilepsy & Creation of Islam

Abbas
Sadeghian Ph.D

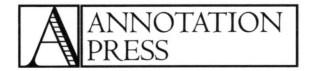

© 2006 by Abbas Sadeghian. All rights reserved

Annotation Press (a division of WinePress Publishing, PO Box 428, Enumclaw, WA 98022) functions only as book publisher. As such, the ultimate design, content, editorial accuracy, and views expressed or implied in this work are those of the author.

No part of this publication may be reproduced, stored in a retrieval system or transmitted in any way by any means—electronic, mechanical, photocopy, recording or otherwise—without the prior permission of the copyright holder, except as provided by USA copyright law.

ISBN 1-59977-002-4
Library of Congress Catalog Card Number: 2005936737

*To the kids of the Middle East,
with the hope of a better tomorrow.*

اسرار ازل را نه تو دانی و نه من
وین حرف معمی نه تو خوانی و نه من
هست از پس پرده گفتگوی من و تو
چون پرده برافتد نه تو مانی و نه من

The secrets eternal neither you know nor I
And answers to the riddle neither you know nor I
Behind the veil there is much talk about us, why
When the veil falls, neither you remain nor I.

        Omar Khayyam

Table of Contents

Map of Arabia XIII
Acknowledgments XV
Introduction XVII

Chapter One—The Time of Ignorance 23
    This chapter describes Muhammad's environment. Fortunately, historians who covered Muhammad's life made an attempt to write about this part of history, which is called Jahiliyah, or "the Time of Ignorance."

Chapter Two—Muhammad's Life Before Islam 41
    Most psychologists would probably agree that we can not know a person without knowing his childhood, which is why this second chapter came into being. Although knowledge of Muhammad's childhood is limited, enough material has been collected to give a reasonable understanding of what occurred during Muhammad's early life.

Chapter Three—The First Revelations 53
   This chapter attempts to report what is known about the events leading to Muhammad's first encounter with the angel Gabriel and the introduction of prophethood to his life. Taken together, the first three chapters are a necessary introduction to the rest of the book.

Chapter Four—Muhammad's Condition 69
   While this chapter regarding Muhammad's condition is my favorite chapter in the book, it was also the most difficult to write. I studied many books to learn of Muhammad's symptoms and reviewed many articles to put the whole premise together. The results were extremely rewarding—as a diagnostician, being able to make the proper diagnosis based on historical facts is extremely valuable.

Chapter Five—Personality Changes: Hyper-Religiosity
   and Sexual Behaviors 89
   Since there was a significant change in Muhammad's behaviors after the onset of the disease—especially after his migration to Medina—I have devoted this chapter to analyzing Muhammad's religiosity and sexual behaviors.

Chapter Six—Personality Changes: Aggression 103
   This chapter focuses on Muhammad's aggressive behaviors. Over the course of these two chapters, the reader will be able to easily see Muhammad's transformation from a passive, small-time merchant to an aggressive, hypersexual, self-proclaimed prophet.

Chapter Seven—The Night Journey: Meeraj 121
   One of the least understood events in Islam is Muhammad's story of his ascension to heaven, which is the source of reference

for the concepts of heaven and hell in Islam. Since the original sources describing heaven and hell are found in other religions, I decided to report the entire dream and explain the historical facts in Zoroastrianism, Christianity, and Islam. This chapter is an attempt to pull these concepts together.

Chapter Eight—Ego Defenses..133
In analyzing any human being's personality, it is necessary to investigate the person's primary ego defenses. The story of Muhammad's encounter with the jinns clearly supports the idea that his primary ego defenses were compensation and rationalization. This chapter tells the story of the jinns and analyzes it in relation to Muhammad's disorder.

Chapter Nine—The Death of the Prophet 141
Last but not least is the issue of Muhammad's death. His last battles, including the conquest of Mecca, lay the groundwork for his final days. It became clear to me while reading about Muhammad and his final sermon that the cause of his death was neurological in origin. Therefore, this final chapter deals with his last four years of his life and the causes of his death.

Appendix I—Complex Partial Seizures...153
The first appendix provides an overview of seizure disorder and its impact on human religious behavior. To prove that Muhammad's claims were caused by his seizures, I felt that it was necessary to explain this condition in detail and provide the rationale that seizures lead to religious delusions. This was a difficult task in the sense that a very technical concept related to diseases of the brain had to be explained in a history book. However, the end result is persuasive and provides the reader with the necessary information to understand the rest of the book

Appendix II—Historical & religious figures suggested in the medical literature to have had epilepsy. 175

The second appendix is a list of other historical and religious figures suspected to have suffered from complex partial seizures.

Bibliography 181

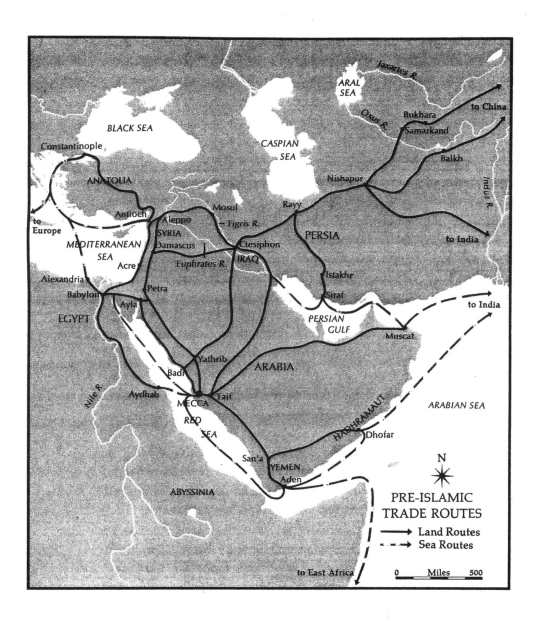

Map of Arabia

Acknowledgements

Writing this book required a lot of help from a lot of friends. I promised every one that their identity would remain anonymous. However, I should take this opportunity and thank every one of them for all of their assistance.

Also, I would like to thank the annotation press and its staff for all of their help and courage which made this book possible.

Introduction

Who am I, and why would I write about Muhammad? I was born and raised in Tehran, Iran. I belonged to the rebellious generation of the 1970s which rose against the rule of Mohammad Reza Shah Pahlavi—the last king of Iran. From a young age I disliked the Iranian government and cooperated with whoever worked against it. In retrospect, I was just a kid and a small pawn in Iranian politics. The end result of our efforts was a big revolution and a huge loss, and the country is, for all practical purposes, gone. The effort to modify Iran from a monarchy to a democracy turned to an exchange from monarchy to theocracy. Since then, I have had a lot of time to reflect and to regret. And there are so many "what ifs."

In 1970, I was accepted at the National University of Iran, where I studied psychology, during this time, I was honored and had the privilege of studying under the supervision of two great American trained psychologists, to whom I shall be indebted forever.

I finished my undergraduate degree in 1975 and was accepted into the London School of Economics and Political Science. I lived in London for one year and studied English, after which time I left London and went to California to study clinical psychology.

It was at about this time that the Iranian revolution began. When the revolution ended, I decided to put politics aside and finish my education. I eventually received my Ph.D. and passed the state boards in psychology. I later became a United States citizen, and I am currently practicing clinical neuropsychology in the United States. I am also an assistant professor of clinical psychology at the Northeastern Ohio Universities College of Medicine. Most of my daily work is diagnostic work-up of patients with neurological disorders. Although my Major has always been psychology, like many other people from Iran, I love Persian literature and world history. I read history books on a daily basis.

During my childhood, I learned of the Prophet Muhammad's life superficially in religious studies classes, and I was acquainted with some of his teachings. Later on during my undergraduate years, while working in Tehran's psychiatric hospitals, I had an eye-opening experience when I met a couple of schizophrenic patients who claimed to be the Messiah. It was not difficult for me to make the connection between these patients' behaviors and what I knew of the behaviors of the prophets. However, with more experience and more education, I realized that a schizophrenic patient does not have the ego strength to tolerate without decompensation the stressors that Muhammad tolerated on his road to becoming a prophet. I decided then that someday, when I had enough knowledge and time, I would study Muhammad's personality in depth, to explore the existence of any psychopathology.

In 1995, I took a detour from practicing clinical psychology to clinical neuropsychology. This detour required additional training, including a two-year postdoctoral study at the New York University's branch of the Fielding Institute. This course of study provided me with the additional knowledge that I needed regarding the workings of the human brain.

While studying the topic of seizure disorder, I came across a nineteenth-century book called *The Blot upon the Brain*. In this book, there was a section in which the author discussed the possibility that the prophet Muhammad suffered from seizure disorder. I began to wonder what sources the author had used to make such claims. As some have a tendency to think that if they discredit Islam they will somehow add to the validity of their own religion, I assumed that the author's hypothesis was based on a religious prejudice.

I did some more research and soon found an article written by Frank Freeman titled *"Differential Diagnosis of the Muhammad the Prophet of Islam"* Although the article did not answer my questions, it rewarded me by pointing me in the direction of other early Islamic sources that could be used in my study. I decided that the time had come to study the original sources of Islam and to educate myself on Muhammad, Islam and the *Quran*.

As I began to study these sources, I soon learned that the people who lived around Muhammad were aware that they were witnessing history in the making, and they did their best to preserve his teachings. In later years, several authors wrote his biography in detail; these biographies, along with the *Quran*, make up the foundations of Islamic theology. Therefore, if I was going to be able to know Muhammad, I had to have access to these ancient books.

Some of the books that I needed were available in English:

1. The *Quran, which* is the holy book of Islam (we will discuss the Quran in much more detail in the course of this book).
2. *Sirat Rasul Allah*, the most famous of biographies of Mohammad originally written by Ibn Ishaq (born A.D. 704 and died A.D. 767), his book was edited and revised by Ibn Hisham (died, A.D. 833 or A.D. 828)
3. *Al Sahih* by Al-Bukhari (died A.D. 892).

Fortunately a couple of these original sources of Islam were available in my native tongue of Persian:

1. *Al-Tabari's* 14 volumes on the history of Islam (died A.D. 839)

2. *Al-Moghazi,* by Al Waghedy (died A.D. 823).

I was also fortunate to find all nine volumes of Al-*Tabaghat Al-cobra* by Ibn Saad (died A.D. 845), written in Arabic. However, since my knowledge of the Arabic language is barely functional, I collected what I found to be useful in these volumes and sent them to international translation centers for proper translation into English. (I kept the translators blind as to what I was doing.). Since I have some knowledge of Turkish, I collected some of the material that I needed from books written in that language.

Along with these original sources, I was also able to obtain a 29-volume interpretation of the *Quran* in Persian written by one of the contemporary ayatollahs in Iran (Ayatollah Nasser Makarem Shirazi).

The combination of these references provided me with the fundamental knowledge of Muhammad's life, the *Quran*, and Islam. I also read most of the contemporary books—pro and against Islam—that I could find in English and Persian to have a better understanding of current analyses of Muhammad's life and Islam.

While researching the life of Muhammad, I studied seizure disorders and their impact on human religiosity. Once the project was reasonably completed, I presented the topic to the department of neuropsychology of New York University. The response was positive and humbling. Up to that point, my intention had been only to print a research article in a psychology journal. However, my colleagues encouraged me to expand the writings and publish them in a book form.

Sword and Seizure is the final product of this research. While writing this book, I had the opportunity to read many books and articles both for and against Muhammad. The pro-Islam books have a tendency to be too nice, minimizing the problems in Muhammad's life and attribute abilities to him that he never had or claimed to have. Some of these books are so far-fetched that they are totally contradictory to Muhammad's teachings (e.g., *Bahar Alanvar* by Majlesi). The books written against Islam are mostly insulting and biased, as they disregard Muhammad's

INTRODUCTION

extraordinary attributes and concentrate on his deficits (e.g., *Muslim Studies* by Goldziher and *Sketches from Eastern History* by Noldeke). However, a common denominator in both sides is a total disregard of the person of Muhammad—why a small-time merchant would pick up such a humongous task, and why was he able to do it.

In this book, I have used the rules of research in psychology to analyze Muhammad and to provide logical answers to the questions surrounding his life. In attempting to achieve this goal, I have done my best to stick to the facts, and I have tried not to permit my own thoughts and prejudices to come into the picture, except on those occasions in which I discovered issues not previously known and felt that I had to report my own thoughts.

Although many books were used in learning about Muhammad, I deliberately limited my reporting of my main arguments to the original sources of Islam and avoided controversial and recent writings. The contemporary sources were mostly used to report well known historical events.

During the course of writing of the book, I felt that it was important to include some information on the neuropsychological aspects of seizure disorder to provide the reader with adequate information regarding the effects of seizure disorder on a person's behavior. However, since putting such a chapter in the middle of a psychohistory book would create a breakdown on the flow of information, I decided to put that section at the end of the book as an appendix .I have tried to make that part of the book as simple as I could. However, I confess that it still is a bit hard to read. The rest of the book is in "black and white" and up to the reader to make his or her conclusions.

One note on the translations used in this book: Since many of the quotes that I have used were brought from Arabic, I tried to report these quotations in both English and Arabic to reduce any possibility of misinterpretation. As previously mentioned, the translations were made by international language centers that were blind to my study.

These translations have also been independently reviewed by various individuals whose native tongue is Arabic.

It should be noted that the copies of the original sources of Islam that were available to me were all twentieth century reprints, and they are recorded in the bibliography for future references.

CHAPTER 1

THE TIME OF IGNORANCE

Our business is to make raids on the enemy, on our neighbor and on our own brother, in case we find none to raid but a brother!
—Hitti 1996

Housed in the Topkapi Museum in Istanbul is a thin-bladed sword called *al-qadib* that resembles a rod. Inscribed in silver on its side are the words: "There is no god but God, Muhammad the messenger of God . . ." Muhammad believed himself to be the messenger of God. But was he, or wasn't he? I do not believe that he was, and therefore the purpose of this book is to provide support for the idea that careful historical examination of the evidence can explain the unusual behavior of people such as Muhammad who claim to be prophets of God.

Human history is filled with thousands of people from many different cultures who have made such grandiose claims. Today's science has revealed that most of these "prophets" were suffering from severe psychiatric problems—mental health professionals in psychiatric hospitals often encounter these individuals. Most of these self-styled prophets were not successful in their endeavors to set themselves up as prophets of God. Muhammad, however, changed the shape of human history. Let's look back and see how this happened.

Arabia at the time of Muhammad

A historical examination of the Prophet Muhammad must begin in the time before his entry onto the world stage. The rough and tumultuous setting into which Muhammad was born and raised did much to shape his personality and later formed the religion of Islam. The time before Muhammad's life-changing interaction with God in the cave of Hira is known to historians as Jahiliyah, which literally means "the Time of Ignorance." It was the time before the world knew the truths that Muhammad would one day reveal.

The Land of Arabia

The Arabian Peninsula is a large, rectangular landmass in southwestern Asia. It comprises some three million square kilometers, an area roughly 10 times the size of modern Italy. The northern end of the peninsula borders the Syrian Desert. The Tigris and Euphrates rivers flow to its northeast. The Persian Gulf joins the Arabian Sea and the Indian Ocean at the Peninsula's northeast, eastern and southern tips. The Red Sea is to the west.

The Arabian Peninsula is divided into three geographical sections: the western section, known as Hejaz (from which Muhammad came); the eastern section, called Najd (home to the peninsula's largest desert, Rub' Al-Khali); and the southern section, Yemen. Hejaz extends from Yemen up the western side of the peninsula to the current Jordanian border. This land has always been rocky, dry and generally inhospitable. Its greatest claim to fame is the two cities that so drastically shaped Muhammad's life and religion: Mecca and Medina.

For a land mass surrounded by so much water, Arabia itself has precious little to spare and lacks fresh water lakes or rivers. The Middle East, and the Arabian Peninsula in particular, has always had an arid

The Time of Ignorance

climate in which water was more precious than gold. Large portions of the country are completely without water. Much of the peninsula is uninhabited desert, the largest of which is Rub' Al-Khali (the "Empty Quarter"). Even today, not more than 22 million people live in the Arabian Peninsula.

However, despite its lack of water, the Arabian Peninsula is not without riches. In Muhammad's day wealth came from gold, silver, and precious stones. But the average citizen of the country had little wealth. Arabs, whether nomadic or stationary, typically scratched out a meager and precarious existence with the aid of camels, horses, birds, dogs, lizards, and ostriches.

Mecca and the Kaaba

Today, Mecca is also one of the most populous cities in Hejaz, with about 150,000 people who call it home. The city sits just 900 feet above sea level and is hidden from distant view by surrounding mountains. Some scientists believe that Mecca sits in the middle of the world's worst geographical climate. Since the land is so salty, it is completely unfit for agriculture. Perhaps it is fortunate for Mecca that early on it became a focal point for tribal religion and commerce.

Many myths have grown up around this famed city. Some claim that Mecca was founded by the prophet Noah, and others claim that the prophet Abraham developed it. Though there is no historical evidence for either claim, the belief persists that Abraham himself was the builder of Mecca's most famous landmark, the Kaaba.

Deep in the heart of a Moslem, there is no sight more sacred than the Kabaa. The Kaaba, which literally means "cube," is a square building made of granite that is located in the center of Mecca near the sacred spring of Zamzam. The Kaaba was built to house one of the most precious artifacts of the ancient Bedouin tribes of the area—the "Black Stone," a meteorite approximately four feet long and a foot wide—which is said to have been placed in the cube by Abraham. Although it is not known when the meteorite may have hit the earth, the spectacle of the fiery rock descending from the heavens undoubtedly had a major impact on the superstitious population.

It is a common human practice that most people like to associate themselves with success. So it is no wonder that some modern Iranian historians believe that the Iranians built the original Kaaba. A similar Kabaa exists in Iran; it is known as the Kaaba of Zartosht, a reference to the prophet of Zoroastrian religion of pre-Islamic Iran. Since it is known that Arabia was periodically under the rule of Iranians, the idea of an Iranian-built Kaaba in Mecca is not terribly far-fetched (Abbasi 2002). Hindus make a similar claim; there is a claim by Indian historians that there was a gold dish hung inside the Kaaba, with "a reference to a king Vikramaditya 'which proves beyond doubt' that the Arabian Peninsula formed a part of his Indian Empire" (P.N. Oak 2003). Whoever the original craftsmen were, it is probable that the Kaaba was modified by various peoples over the course of history in order to accommodate their particular faiths and worship needs.

As the region's most holy shrine, the Kaaba became home to a variety of treasured artifacts. Some 360 idols or effigies of the gods—one for each day of the Sumerian religion's calendar and five for the days for pilgrimage (*hajj*)—were housed inside the building. People came from across the peninsula to walk around the shrine, enjoy the sanctuary of its violence-free zone, and pay homage to the stone and the idols brought there for safekeeping.

Religions in Mecca

While the pagans made up the largest religious group in Mecca during Jahiliyah, they were by no means a cohesive group. The variations of paganism represented were many and complex. A large number of ancient Arabs turned their eyes skyward for objects of worship. The well-known Arab historian Kalbi, in his 10-volume epistle on the subject, writes that the tribe of Bani Malih worshipped the *jinns* (or demons); the Tribe of

The Time of Ignorance

Homair worshipped the sun; the tribe of Tamiam worshipped the *dabran*, a cluster of five stars; the tribe of Laman worshipped the Greek goddess Venus; and the Tey worshipped Sohail (Sobhani 1994, 1:43).

The pagans created a multitude of idols, which they adored and feared. They decorated these images with gold and silver and hung them with wooden carvings. Before any major decision was made, the worshipper consulted these idols in a sort of ancient tea leaf ritual. After asking a question of the idol, the worshipper plucked an answer from a pile of wooden carvings, reading either "yes" or "no." It was not unusual for the devout pagan to bring sacrifices and bow to his idols many times each day. When the tribes were away from their idols, they gathered beautiful stones and constructed temporary desert altars. More often, idols were brought along on trips and into battle. It was an honor for a person just to be chosen to help bear the tribal idols.

Three of the ancient idols that were considered superior to all others were Lat, Manat, and Uzzah. Mecca's major tribe, the Ghouraish, believed these idols to be the three daughters of God, and their exalted status afforded them special treatment. A shrine of beautiful white stones was erected to Lat in the city of Taief. Manat, the goddess of fortune and future, was enshrined in Qudayd. The most popular of them all, however, was the shrine of Uzzah ("mighty and powerful"), which was located in the famous village of Nakhleh located somewhere between Mecca and Medina.

Idols weren't the only sacred items in the lives of these ancient people. In addition to worshipping the idols themselves and the various heavenly bodies, it was not unusual for tribal people of the day to find religious significance in stones, dates, dust and wood. With so many different families and tribes paying homage to such a wide variety of idols (and even household gods), it is not surprising that tempers often flared between peoples in the name of religion. Tribal wars and major bloodshed were not uncommon. It was a time of uneasy faith.

In addition to the various pagan tribes, other world religions were also represented in Arabia during Jahiliyah. The people of Persia (to the northeast of the peninsula in current Iran) were Zoroastrian, possessing their own bible (Avesta) and prophet (Zartosht, or Zarathustra as the Greek called him and as popularized by Nietzsche). Arabic towns to the northeast absorbed some of this religious culture, but many remained skeptical of the major religious systems and clung fiercely to their independence.

Commerce with Byzantium also brought early Christianity to the region (Armstrong 1992). Some of the tribes in Arabia had absorbed the monotheistic teachings of the prophet Abraham, whom they called Hanaffiya. Additionally, Judaism was practiced in Arabia, and many Jewish practices were adopted even by non-Jews. Historians have found that Arabic people of various faiths incorporated Jewish ceremonies and fasting into their daily religious lives.

It has been suggested that the cause of the revengeful fights of Jahiliyah was the belief that at death the soul departed the body in the form of an owl-like creature known as Hameh. Once freed from the body, the Hameh was believed to sit next to its departed host and wail mournfully. After burial, the tomb became home to the disenfranchised Hameh. Although the Hameh might occasionally leave the tomb to collect information on its living relatives, it would typically spend a peaceful eternity watching over its former host—that is, unless the host had died of unnatural causes. Unavenged murder meant the Hameh was forced to scream forever, demanding the blood of the killer. Since only revenge would quiet the raging Hameh, wars between tribes and smaller family groups (clans) were constant and bitter and could last for centuries. To ancient Arabs, war was a fact of life and a matter of honor. Tribal leaders were expected to keep vendettas in order to prove and preserve the tribe's honor and respect (Sobhani 1994, 1:46).

Medina

The other significant city in Hejaz (and to the life of Muhammad) was Medina. Originally called Yathreb, Medina was the next largest city to

The Time of Ignorance

Mecca. Unlike Mecca, however, the improved climate and soil made Medina more agriculturally sound. Hence, it enjoyed a relatively hospitable climate, boasting many an oasis and more plentiful water.

Though first populated by various Arabic tribes, Mecca and Medina began to attract people from outside the peninsula, particularly from nearby Syria. Believing that the Messiah would come to the Arabian Peninsula, some Jewish tribes relocated to Mecca or Medina. (The Roman conquest of their homeland in the first and second centuries A.D. was an added incentive to move.) These Jewish tribes often had Arabic names, and although the most significant of them stayed in Medina, other lesser Jewish tribes eventually spread throughout the peninsula. In time, a hierarchy of servitude emerged. For example, Arabic tribes native to Yathreb, such as the Ous and Khazraj, ended up working for the transplanted Jewish farmers and merchants.

YEMEN

To the south of Hejaz sits Yemen. Largely because of its access to water, Yemen was a famous region in the ancient world. The Queen of Sheba, is said to have hailed from the capital city of Yemen, now known as Sana'a. Yemen was an Arabic success story. Advanced methods of irrigation and agriculture gave rise to greater wealth, which, in turn, made larger and more ornate buildings possible. Even today, the castles and fine architecture found throughout Yemen are a testimony to its historical significance. Yemen became a popular area for many tribes, who brought with them their various religions: paganism, Judaism, Christianity, and Zoroastrianism. The diversity sparked wars, making the region well known for its instability.

Although the major powers outside the peninsula courted the leaders of Yemen, even the region's ports, farms and more sophisticated culture were not enough to entice these powers to attempt to conquer Arabia. The fact remained that most of the region was dry and unfriendly, populated by nomadic tribes who drifted through the deserts in search of fertile grazing land for their camels or for other tribes to raid. There were few cities outside of Mecca and Medina, no laws, hundreds of different dialects and pagan religions, and no centralized government. With the exception of Yemen, the region had no particular strategic significance, and little wealth. Small wonder then that the far more advanced Iran to the northeast of the peninsula had no interest in the region, nor did the Eastern Roman Empire of the Byzantines. For much of recorded history, the Arabian Peninsula was the most unwanted piece of territory in the Middle East. These other civilizations wanted nothing more than to keep the Arabs in their place by whatever means necessary.

The Persian Gulf

The Persian Gulf is a body of water that extends from the eastern edge of the Arabian Peninsula to the Strait of Hormous, where it flows into the Sea of Amman and the Indian Ocean. The Gulf takes its title from the ancient Greek name for Iran (Persia literally means "Land of the Pars," the most dominant Aryan tribe in the area at the time).

Because of poor navigational systems and badly built ships, ancient merchants preferred to travel on land as much as possible, making the shortcut through the Persian Gulf as vital then as it is now. Spices and goods that were brought from India to Rome and the rest of the ancient world had to be transported through the Strait of Hormous to what is now the city of Basra on the northwest tip of the Gulf. From there, goods could be taken by caravan through Iran to Syria and into the west. It was a lucrative business for Arab tribes, many of whom were hired in a protective capacity for the caravans.

Then, as now, the Persian Gulf was strategic. Not only was it an important route for transport, but its warm, shallow waters also provided an excellent breeding ground for pearls. Although it was dangerous and difficult work, pearl diving provided a major source of revenue for the Gulf region. Today, the gulf island of Bahrain remains one of the world's best pearl hunting grounds. Most of the region's rich oil reservoirs lie close to the Gulf, and 60 percent of the modern world's oil is transported through the Gulf and the Strait of Hormous.

LIFE IN ARABIA

Restlessness was par for the course in ancient Arabia. Nomadic tribes had become so out of necessity, constantly forced to search for water, better soil and grazing land. When rain came to a region, tribal people with their flocks and camels would flood into the area, consuming whatever water and vegetation they could find until it was gone. The region's precious water wells, scattered throughout the peninsula, were a major source of conflict among tribes, many of whom preferred death over relinquishing their claim on life-giving water.

THE CAMEL

There was arguably nothing more significant to ancient Arabian life than the camel, which was domesticated about 2,000 years before the time of Muhammad. The camel's ability to store water and traverse the deserts at tremendous speed (not to mention its milk, a mainstay of the nomadic diet) made the nomadic life possible. Camels are not casual drinkers like horses or cattle or even humans—they drink slowly, but they deliberately consume enormous quantities of water. Camels then preserve this water in their blood, which allows them to travel up to 10 days without drinking. In addition to storing water in their blood, camels also keep a reserve supply in their stomachs. (Water is not stored in the hump as is sometimes thought; however, the hump is composed of fatty tissue, which provides the camel with a source of calories for long desert journeys.)

Even today, desert travelers faced with a desperate shortage of water might tap into that reserve by actually sucking water out of the camel's stomach: "There is hardly a member of the tribe who has not on some occasion drunk water from a camel's paunch. In time of emergency either an old camel is killed or a stick is thrust down its throat to make it vomit water. If the camel has been watered within a day or two, the liquid is tolerably drinkable" (Hitti 1996). Times change, but the dependency of man on the camel does not. Many camels have saved the lives of their human traveling companions in this way.

Without the camel, the desert could not be conceived of as a habitable place. It is the nomad's nourisher, his vehicle of transportation, and his medium of exchange. The dowry of the bride, the price of blood, the profit of gambling, and the wealth of a sheikh—all are computed in terms of camels. The camel is the Bedouin's constant companion, his alter ego and his foster parent. He drinks its milk instead of water, which he spares for the cattle; he feasts on its flesh; he covers himself with its skin; he makes his tent of its hair. He uses its dung as fuel and its urine as a hair tonic and medicine (when used as shampoo, it leaves an odor on the hair corresponding to perfume; when used on the face, it provides a layer of oil serviceable as a protection against insect bites). To the Bedouin, the camel is more than "the ship of the desert"; it is the special gift of Allah (Hitti 1996).

Without camels, life for man in the desert would have been just about nonexistent. Before the domestication of the camel, most Arabs were forced to endure a stationary existence, which (depending on their particular location and access to water) could be extraordinarily difficult, if not impossible.

Farming Tribes and the Ghazw

Not all ancient Arabs were nomadic. Some were able to establish and maintain small farms. It has been postulated that nomadic tribes were "followed step by step by pioneering farmers who settled in the oases and ... made the desert bloom" (Armstrong 1992). Nomadic and farming tribes established a tenuous mutual dependence. Some nomads, who were generally more skillful warriors, would provide protection and foreign goods in exchange for a portion of the harvest. These desert farms could easily fall prey to nomadic tribes who accepted as a matter of course that they could raid the camps or homes of their enemies with impunity. Raids were not even frowned upon among the tribes, provided the raiders were not robbing members of their own clan or tribe.

The raid or *ghazw* (corrupted into "razzia"), otherwise considered a form of brigandage, is raised by the economic and social conditions of desert life to the rank of a national institution. It lies at the base of the economic structure of Bedouin pastoral society. In desert land, where the fighting mood is a chronic mental condition, raiding is one of the few manly occupations. Christian tribes, too, practiced it. Such life is best described in these two verses: "Our business is to make raids on the enemy, on our neighbor and on our own brother, in case we find none to raid but a brother!" (Hitti 1996).

> According to the rules of the game—*ghazw* was a sort of national sport—no blood should be shed except in cases of extreme necessity. *Ghazw* does help to a certain extent to keep down the number of mouths to feed, though it does not actually increase the sum total of available supplies. A weaker tribe or a sedentary settlement on the borderland could buy protection by paying tribute to the stronger tribe. (Hitti 1996)

STATUS OF WOMEN

Without clan protection, the life of an individual Arab was worthless. At the same time, the existence of the tribe was dependant on the total number of existing men. A person who had many brothers and male cousins would automatically have more power within the clan than one who did not, and the same held true for a clan or a tribe. This is the primary reason for the preference of having a son rather than a daughter: boys were assets for the family, clan, and tribe; girls were a liability. This fact, one way or another, is still true among people of the Middle East.

If the life of Arab men was difficult, the life of the average ancient Arab woman must have been close to unbearable. A woman was considered a man's belonging and could be traded, bought, or sold at the will of her husband. Although a man had to agree to pay off his wife should he ever decide to leave her, most could avoid the practice by accusing the woman of infidelity. Violence and battery was another common way for a man to get rid of his wife without paying.

Women were perceived as "pots" for the carrying of fetuses and did not stand to inherit anything from their husbands. On the contrary, a man's son would inherit his wives upon his death and could do with them what he wished. Widows who wanted to remarry had to pay off their former husband's son for the privilege. Even cattle were prized more highly than women, since cattle tended to retain their value with age. Female infants were buried alive at times so that the family did not have to deal with them.

The Muruwah

Arab men prided themselves on their ability to be good warriors. Their actions were ruled by a sort of ancient Arab chivalry, known as *muruwah*, which prompted them to take vengeance on enemies, patiently endure suffering, and protect the tribe's weakest members. Although *muruwah* is often translated by English scholars as "manliness," in Arabic its meaning is more complex and extensive. Each tribe prided itself on its own special brand of *muruwah*, which was believed to be inherited by blood (Armstrong 1992).

Ancient Arabs had their own set of scruples. On the whole, history shows them to have been an honest and straightforward people, true to their word, and willing to fight and die to protect their clans, families, and beliefs. Horseback riding was a favorite activity. They were courageous in battle and ruthless in conquest. In war, winning tribes typically decapitated their defeated enemies, confiscated their belongings, and made slaves of their women and children, thus making it less likely that they themselves would later fall victim to a vengeful attack.

Arabic Diet

The Arabic diet was as rough and precarious as the rest of their lives. Camel milk was a stable source of nutrition, as were the desert animals they managed to hunt. Lizards and grasshoppers were delicacies. From the farming Arabs, nomadic people could obtain such supplements as dates and wheat for making bread. Dates were one of the most desired foods in the Middle East and could also be obtained from palm trees, the greatest gift of the desert.

Commerce

Among the Bedouin tribes, even bitter enemies would lay down their arms and do business together in Mecca, where ancient Arabs had devised a brilliant arrangement to encourage trade. Drawing on the sacredness of the Kaaba, the house of the gods, fighting was forbidden in or around the sacred site. In addition, fighting ceased for four months out of the year across Arabia so that tribes could safely travel to Mecca to pay homage to their favorite idols and buy and sell goods. The practice was so deeply ingrained among ancient Arabs that the prophet Muhammad eventually incorporated some of these ideas and rituals into his own teachings.

But not all Arabs were content to be kept on their peninsula, alternately trading and fighting amongst themselves. Some gazed across the border into Persia and Byzantium and, wanting what they saw, eventually left the peninsula to plunder and pillage their richer northern neighbors. When chased, the tribes (who were accustomed to life in the harsh Arabian climate) simply took off for the most inhospitable areas of the desert and waited there until their pursuers gave up.

Both Persia and Rome hired Arab tribes to live in their border cities to protect them against the more aggressive nomadic Arabs. (These tribes, similar to those who escorted caravans of merchandise, apparently had a knack for protection.) The most famous of these border towns was Hiran, located on the banks of the Euphrates at the southern edge of Persia. The arrangement seemed to work well until, during Muhammad's boyhood, the Persian Emperor, Khosro II (also known as Khosro Parviz) killed the leader of the tribe protecting Hiran. Persia quickly lost the protection of the Arabian tribes, leaving their border cities vulnerable to invading forces. Historians believe that this one event helped pave the way for the rapid expansion of the religion of Islam just a few years later.

Travel

Trade routes, rough and difficult as they were, eventually became ancient roads. Taking a trade caravan across such roads necessitated a great deal of preparation. Of course, travelers had to carry an ample supply of water packed on top of camels. They often also brought horses, which were faster and useful for fighting should the need arise. Depending on their origins and familiarity with the region, caravans typically relied on local guides to traverse the huge, empty expanses of sand. Such caravans might require their own security forces, which varied from just a few armed men to a force of several tribes. Only those who had spent their lives in the desert had even the slimmest chance of success in such a field.

To avoid the intensity of the desert sun, caravans usually traveled from 3 A.M. until noon, stopping at the ancient equivalent of a motel called a *manzel*, or *caravansara* ("house of the caravan"). In wealthier areas or in places ruled by a central government, a *manzel* might be a decent building adjacent to a spring or well. In poorer areas, staying at the local *manzel* could be taking your life into your hands. Instead of the traditional night's rest, the caravan would move on quickly from such a place, just hoping to avoid getting caught up in any local unrest.

Learning

During this period, there was much work being done in Rome and Persia by Christian, Zoroastrian and Mythraistic theologians in the area of scientific discovery and other fields of learning. The universities of Alexandria in Egypt and Jondy Shapour in Persia were famous for their achievements at this time. The works of Greek philosophers and scien-

The Time of Ignorance

tists had been translated to local languages, and scholars were eagerly adding to this body of knowledge. Many scholars believe that Persia was the strongest country in the world and that Rome was the richest.

In Arabia, however, there was an almost total absence of scientific discovery, schools, universities or learning of any kind during this time. It is said that at the time of Muhammad there were only 17 people living in Mecca who could read and write. There was not even an attempt to import any of the new knowledge from Rome and Persia until hundreds of years after Christ. The difficulties of tribal life and the lack of central government made simple existence challenging enough for the Arabs.

Although many of the poor, hard living ancient Arabs could neither read nor write, they valued the spoken and written Arabic language, which was not unlike modern Arabic. They placed a special value on poetry. Well-spoken tribal members memorized and recited epic poems celebrating the courageous victories of the tribe. These poems were an elaborate record of the tribe's history and provided a source of hope for its future. In fact, they were considered so important to tribal life that the ability to compose and recite inspired poetry was believed to be a sign of divine favor. Such poets were thought to be possessed by a spirit and imbued with mystical powers.

The love of poetry and the spoken language not only provided a rich oral history for future generations of Arabs but also made for good entertainment on hot desert nights. Poetry was valued so highly that poems deemed to be the very best would be hung in the Kaaba. These poems were called the *Al Moaallaghat* ("Hanged Ones"), and although many centuries have passed, these early works of literature are still cherished throughout the Arabic world.

So even though ancient Arabs were not making significant developments in science during this period, Arab intellectuals made major contributions with their poems. The greatest poets were able to sell their poetry extolling various conquerors, tribal leaders, and wealthy individuals to the subjects of those poems. Consequently, although poetry itself was highly prized, the profession of poet was not considered honorable.

MEDICAL PRACTICES AND SUPERSTITIONS

Superstitions and the rituals surrounding them were another means by which pre-Islamic Arabs tried to exert some control over their fragile existence. Long, dark desert nights could be frightening, and contact with other tribes was often scarce. Communication between the scattered groups was impossible. The need to appease the gods, goddesses, and demons that ruled their fates was a way of life for these ancient nomads.

Medicine consisted primarily of ridding the afflicted person of demons. The term *majanoon* (or "mentally ill"), coined during ancient times, persists today in meaning afflicted by *jinns,* or demons. Because demons were thought to be ousted with dirt, schizophrenics were given a necklace made of the contaminated clothes of the dead. Victims of snake or scorpion bites were adorned with protective gold and silver, since it was believed that in such cases low-level metals like copper or tin would be deadly. A person bitten by a mad dog was treated by rubbing that person's own blood (from another cut) on the bite to prevent the psychosis that such a bite could cause. Gathering food from various tribal households and feeding it to the tribe's dogs could treat a child with a blister on his mouth or face.

Skin diseases were thought to be the result of the victim killing a snake or scorpion that belonged to the demons. To make amends and promote healing, a clay camel was fashioned, adorned with grain and dates, and put it in the pathways of the snakes. If the food was tampered with the next day, the demons were thought to have been appeased—a sure sign that the afflicted person would recover. In one of the stranger superstitions, people entering a village that was rife with cholera or some other epidemy would spend a few moments standing by the city gates braying like a donkey. Doing this 10 times was thought to protect the person entering the city against illness.

Because drought was always a problem, one superstition held that irate bulls could persuade the heavens to open up. During drought years, tribal people would take bulls to the top of the nearest hill, tie pieces of dry wood to their tails, and light the wood on fire. It was thought that the screaming, flailing animal would replicate the sound of thunder and thereby stir up a storm. Wearing clothes inside out was also believed to help one find his way when lost in the desert (Sobhani 1994, 1:58).

Sorcerers and Magicians

In a society in which religious ideas were wrapped up in primitive superstitions, sorcerers had an easy opening. Ancient Arabian sorcerers were typically half delusional and half devious. These charlatans devoted their lives to devising complex methods for treating disease with various primitive materials. They were frequently engaged to fight demons and rid the afflicted of goblins and *jinns*.

The relationship between the general public and its sorcerers was again love-hate. People tended to devaluate and distrust magicians, even as they turned to them for help. It has been reported and there are several Hadith (stories from the life of the Prophet) that claim Muhammad had a total distaste for poets and sorcerers. As a righteous man, Muhammad believed himself to be above such people. His moralistic view of the world would have prevented him from even the thought of engaging in poetic work.

In short, the time and place that Muhammad was born was just about as bad as it could get. It was the furthest from civilization, and the harshest environment in which to live. At the same time, it was ripe for a change, as Arabs could easily see that their lives were so different to people of other lands who had so much more and lived so much better. They desperately needed a man to pull them out of that burning furnace.

CHAPTER 2

MUHAMMAD'S LIFE BEFORE ISLAM

أَلَمْ يَجِدْكَ يَتِيمًا فَآوَى

Did He not find you an orphan and give you shelter?
—The Quran, 93:6

Muhammad was born in Mecca, but the exact date of his birth is the subject of some debate among scholars. Most agree that he was born on Monday the twelfth of Rabi-1, the Year of the Elephant (Ibn Ishaq, 69), which is August 20, 570 A.D. by the Roman calendar (Wintle 2003). Muhammad was raised in the part of the Middle East that we now know as Saudi Arabia.

The difficulty of pinpointing Muhammad's exact date of birth is exacerbated by the ancient Arabian practice of starting a new calendar when there was a major event. The year that the major event occurred would become Year One, and the years would then be numbered in succession until the next major event. The year that the king of Ethiopia invaded Arabia riding on an elephant was known as Aam Olfil, or the "Year of the Elephant." The significance of this event made that year the first in a new calendar, and many historians have confirmed that Muhammad was born during that time.

Mecca at the Time of Muhammad

Before examining the specifics of Muhammad's birth, it is important to first understand the setting into which he was born. In addition to being a holy city, Mecca was home to an important well (known as Zamzam) and therefore a vital stopping place for caravans traversing the peninsula. In the ancient Middle East, caravans traveling between Yemen and Syria typically selected a number of stopping places during their journey. These cities were picked primarily on the availability of sufficient water for the travelers and their animals, access to other provisions the travelers might need, and for reasons of security (cities that proved to be troublesome from a security standpoint would be eliminated from the travel plans on the next trip). It was in a city's best interest to cater to these caravans. Mecca took up the challenge. The fact that it was a water city made it especially appealing to caravans.

During the four months of the year in which fighting was forbidden on the peninsula, groups of people from various tribes would travel to Mecca for a fair. This was a time of worship, commerce, and tourism. The buying and selling of slaves, drinking, gambling, and other types of cavorting were rampant among the warriors during this time off. Of course, such activities also called for an ample supply of water.

The business of making sure that the camels, travelers and merchants were supplied with the water they needed fell to Muhammad's family. The family belonged to the tribe of Ghouraish, and Muhammad's clan was the Bani Hashim. Muhammad's grandfather, Abdul-Mottaleb, was actually the keeper of the famous Zamzam well. The well itself was actually more like a large pool, and overseeing it was one of the most important jobs in the city. Abdul-Mottaleb relied on his sons and other members of his clan for help in this job. His status as the chief caretaker for the well earned him great prestige in religious circles as well as power, wealth, and connections (Sobhani 1994).

Muhammad's Childhood

Abdul-Mottaleb had several wives and many sons. One of these sons, Abdullah, married a woman named Amina and fathered Muhammad. There are many legends regarding Amina's pregnancy and Muhammad's naming (Al-Tabari, Persian translation, 1990) however they are mostly made up stories. What we know for a fact is that the name "Muhammad" was not a very popular name at that time (Sobhani 1994); while currently it is the most popular name in the world.

Abdullah died in Medina on his way back from a trip to Syria before his son Muhammad was born. As was customary at the time, Muhammad spent the first few weeks with his mother, after which his care was entrusted to his grandfather. It was typical in Arabia during this time to remove young children from the city in order to protect them from deadly diseases (such as cholera) that tended to crop up in places where there were densely packed groups of people living with their animals. Instead, children were given to the care of a desert tribe until they were older and thus had a greater chance of survival in the cities (Armstrong 1992). This custom is still observed among many well-to-do families in Arabia for the same reasons.

Muhammad was cared for by two nannies. The first nanny was Soiebeh, a slave of the family, who suckled the baby for several months. The second nanny was Halimeh, from the tribe of Bani Saad, who took Muhammad out of Mecca to the desert and raised him for the first five years of his life (Sobhani 1994). The people of the Bani Saad are famous for being especially articulate and for having an excellent command of the Arabic language. It has been postulated that the seeds of Muhammad's great knowledge of Arabic were planted during the first few years that he spent with the Bani Saad.

The introduction of little Muhammad into Halimeh's household had a major impact on her family. Halimeh had a son of her own, whom she could not nurse. She claimed that she was so poor and hungry that her milk had simply dried up, leaving her tiny son to cry out in the night from hunger. But when she assumed the care of Muhammad, things began to change. Halimeh claimed that her breasts began to fill with milk again, enough for both Muhammad and her own child. The family's old female camel, which had also not given any milk for ages, suddenly began producing again and provided the whole family with the nourishment that they had long been without. Even Halimeh's donkey transformed from an animal that could barely move to one that could travel faster than a horse (Ibn Ishaq, P71).

Many Islamic writers, both ancient and modern, recount numerous other miracles that occurred upon the birth of Muhammad. In his book *Tarikh Gozidh*, the Islamic writer Hamdolah Moustofi claims that when Muhammad was born, thousands of new stars appeared in the skies. All the idols in the Kaaba broke into pieces and the fire in the Fire Shrine of Pars in Iran suddenly died. It should be noted that the Fire Shrine of Pars was one of the most important shrines of the Zoroastrian religion and had been watched over by hundreds of caretakers for centuries. As a testament to their hatred of Iranian kings, many other writers also claim that a big crack appeared in the dome in the castle of the king of Persia and the ceiling collapsed (the ruins of the castle are still in Iraq with an intact dome). Some Iranian clergymen at the time reportedly had dreams that their camels were getting weaker while the Arabic camels grew fat and healthy (Mostofi, reprinted 1988). Ironically, Muhammad himself never made such claims and requested that people not ask him for miracles.

These strange events didn't stop with Muhammad's birth. In another famous story, when Muhammad was about three years old, his cousin is said to have run, breathless, into the house to report that two men had come and removed part of Muhammad's body. Alarmed, Muhammad's nanny, Halimeh, ran from the house to find Muhammad badly shaken by the incident. Muhammad is said to have told her that two men in white clothes (believed to be angels) laid him down, opened his breast, played with his heart, and removed something dark from his chest. Muhammad and his cousin said that the men healed the wound and then left, although Halimeh could find no scar. As the story goes, Halimeh was so frightened by the event that she took the young boy back to his mother in Mecca (Armstrong 1992). Since it is widely accepted that Muhammad lived in the desert among the Bani Saad until he was five, the story is probably not accurate. Some authors have postulated that the episode was actually Muhammad's first seizure. However, like so many stories surrounding Muhammad's birth and childhood, this also is unlikely.

Muhammad was brought back to his mother, Amina, in Mecca when he was five years old. Some reports indicate that he was returned because Halimeh feared that Muhammad had been afflicted by demons, and she wanted him to be with his mother. Amina got angry at the accusation and promptly took him back. Soon after arriving in Mecca, Amina took Muhammad to Medina to visit family and see the burial site of Abdullah, Muhammad's father. On the way home from Medina, Amina became sick and died (Sobhani 1994).

The loss of his father and now his mother at such a young age had a major and lasting impact on Muhammad, who was now once again under the supervision of his grandparents. As he grew up, Muhammad talked at length with his friends about being an orphan. The *Quran* reflects his strong feelings on the issue—on more than 20 occasions, the *Quran* prohibits the abuse of orphans and extols the virtues of taking in and caring for orphaned children.

Under the care of his grandfather, Abdul-Mottaleb, Muhammad began taking odd jobs that were available to boys his age. His primary job as a child was a shepherd. He cared for camels and cattle on the outskirts of Mecca and earned a small wage. But his secure and simple life was short-lived; when Muhammad was eight years old, his grandfather died at the age of 80. It has been reported that Abdul-Mottaleb emphasized on his deathbed that the family should take care of Muhammad. However, it has also been said that Abdul-Mottaleb was mute during the last days of his life. Whatever the truth, Muhammad was once again orphaned and alone in the world.

Eventually, Muhammad was sent to live with his uncle Abu Taleb, who was from the same mother as Abdullah Muhammad's father (Ibn Ishaq, P179). Although Muhammad's clan was relatively rich, Abu Taleb himself was not wealthy. He was, however, famous for his generosity. To help make ends meet in his new family, Muhammad continued to work as a shepherd.

When Muhammad was 12 years old, Abu Taleb decided to travel to Syria on business and allowed Muhammad to tag along (Al-Tabari Persian translation, 1990, 3:829). The trip took them to the city of Bastra in the southern part of Syria. Some historians claim that Muhammad encountered a number of Christian and Jewish clergy during this trip and that they recognized he would grow up to become the Prophet. This scenario is extremely unlikely, because Muhammad himself was 40 years old before the first thought about being a prophet ever came to his mind. In any event, Muhammad's first trip to Syria was a bright spot in his young life and gave him his first real opportunity to see new places, meet foreign people, and learn of other religions.

When Muhammad was between 15 and 20 years old, he got his first taste of battle. A brutal and greedy tribe had violated the four-month prohibition on fighting, instigating the War of Fejar, which lasted for four years. Once first blood was drawn, the need for vengeance overshadowed other time-honored rules, and fighting ensued. Although Muhammad himself is not believed to have fought on the battlefield, he supplied soldiers with arrows, collecting them from the battlefield and returning them to the fighting men (Ibn Saad 1990, 1:101). Some historians, however, believe that Muhammad did, in fact, participate during this war as an archer. In either case, the War of Fejar gave Muhammad the opportunity to gain some knowledge of the techniques and tactics of battle. In the end, both sides agreed to settle the conflict by counting up the number of dead. The clan with the fewest losses would reimburse the other tribe for its dead. Muhammad's side, which counted 20 fewer deaths than their rival, paid the blood money, and the war ended.

Muhammad preferred the quiet of the countryside to the stressful life of the city. He made only a few trips to Mecca, preferring instead to spend the nights among his sheep, absorbing the clean, fresh desert air and gazing at the magnificent desert night sky. The desert's pure air lends the sky a depth and richness that can be seen in few other places. The sky actually appears to be multi-dimensional, and many stars are visible. Faced with such an awe-inspiring sight, it is hard to imagine that Muhammad did not spend time pondering his existence and the origins of life.

Muhammad's Adult Life

When he was 25 years old, Muhammad married Khadijeh, a prominent woman in Mecca. This relationship was to have an enormous psychological impact on Muhammad's life. At a time when most men married before age 20 and most girls were married by age 16, Muhammad's situation was unusual from the start. It was made even more unusual by the fact that he was probably a virgin when he wed (Mostofi, reprinted 1988).

There is very little known about Muhammad's life at this time, which makes it difficult to account for his late introduction into the world of male-female relationships. (Most books on Muhammad simply skip over this part of his life.)

Certainly, the lack of a father and the loss of his mother at such a young age would have had an enormous impact on the boy's psychological development. Muhammad had no brothers or sisters and, having never lived for long with his own family, probably missed out entirely on the warmth and love of a normal parent. Childhood friendships, grandfathers, uncles, and cousins are poor substitutes for a mother's love. Given the myriad of losses in his life, it is not surprising that Muhammad was plagued by fears and insecurities. His unusual first marriage is likely to have been a byproduct of those childhood events.

Although Khadijeh was Muhammad's first wife, she had been married twice before. The rich, older widow had employed Muhammad to travel to Syria to conduct some business for her. Upon his return, she was so impressed with his honesty (not to mention the profits he had earned for her) that she expressed a desire to marry him. With the mediation of some family members and after some tribal negotiations, Khadijeh and Muhammad were married. Some believe that she was 40 years old, but it has also been reported that Khadijeh bore Muhammad six or eight children (Al-Tabari Persian translation 1990,4:1288), which would probably have made her younger than 40 at the time of their marriage. In any case, Muhammad apparently did not care about the age difference. His devotion was unquestioned and he took no other wives during their marriage. Even after Khadijah's death, Muhammad spoke of her with great respect and love. With her constant emotional support (quite likely the first he had ever known) and acceptance of his claims to be the prophet of Allah, Khadijeh paved the way for Muhammad's transformation.

MUHAMMAD THE HONEST

Because Muhammad's devout followers (who naturally portray him in the best possible light) have written most of the accounts of his life and personality, it is difficult to get a clear picture of his true character. It is rare to find a single negative attribute in any book on the Prophet. We do know that his behavior during this time distinguished him among his fellow Arabs. He was called Muhammad al-Amin (Sobhani 1994), which literally means "Muhammad, the trustworthy and honest". At a time when wars were waged among tribes over minuscule amounts of money, the fact that Muhammad was singled out as *Amin* is a testament to his efforts to live an honorable life. In fact, he had few of the attributes typically aspired to by other young men of the time. He was not a noted sword fighter or even a sword maker. Neither was he an accomplished horseman. When future generations asked Ali, the Prophet's cousin, about Muhammad's looks, Ali said:

Our prophet was not short nor was he tall. He had big head and very full beard. He was big boned with strong arms and legs. His face was reddish, and he had a hairy chest, while walking he leaned forward, like a person who is walking down hill. Never before and never after I have seen anybody like him. (Al-Tabari, Persian translation, 1990, 4:1307)

By all accounts, this simple shepherd stood out among his fellow men by following a path of righteousness and goodness. Muhammad was clearly intelligent; by his wits alone, he had managed to elevate himself from a poor dispossessed orphan to the husband of one of the tribe's wealthiest widows. The miraculous nature of that achievement was not lost on his clansmen. Some point to this ability of Muhammad to wrestle success from almost certain failure as proof of divine intervention in his life. (Certainly, those who are familiar with the plight of orphans in the Middle East can appreciate the marked contrast between Muhammad and others in his situation.) Muhammad clearly believed that God had a hand in his success. Even the *Quran* makes reference to his orphanhood and to the fact that God had taken care of him:

ألمْ يَجِدْكَ يَتِيمًا فَآوَى

Did He not find you an orphan and give you shelter? (93:6)

Muhammad's keen intellect also made him an excellent negotiator. The following story proves his problem solving skills. When burglars made off with gold and idols from the Kaaba (which was not a strong structure and didn't even have a roof), the keepers of the Kaaba decided to build something more secure. They decided that the new Kaaba needed to be bigger and have a door that would lock. To build the larger building, the keepers needed plenty of wood, which was a rare commodity in the desert—most homes were built of clay or brick. Fortunately, a wooden ship had run aground in the nearby port city of Jeddah. Here was an instant source of the needed wood. So, in a short time the builders of the new Kaaba had it ready once again to house Mecca's treasures, the chief of which is the Black Stone.

It was an honor just to touch the Black Stone, let alone pick it up and move it. Four different tribes laid claim to the honor of replacing the Black Stone. These tribes were on the brink of war over the matter when Muhammad intervened. He wisely suggested a compromise: The four leaders would lay the Stone in the center of a blanket and each one would hold a corner of the blanket, thereby sharing the honor. In appreciation for his wisdom, the grateful tribal leaders granted Muhammad the ultimate honor of picking up the stone to place it on the blanket (Ibn Ishaq, P86).

Being a religious man from a religious family, Muhammad was said to be especially fond of the Kaaba. Muhammad's family even took a turn as keepers of the Kaaba. Muhammad would indulge in many of the rituals surrounding the Kaaba at the time, including the practice of walking around the building (circumbulition), meditating, and praying to the gods inside (Ibn Ishaq, P86). Although he was clearly pious, most of Muhammad's biographers report that he followed the religion of Abraham, a monotheistic faith that focused on God alone (*Hanaffiya*). Muhammad was also exposed to Judeo-Christian ideas as a result of having regular contact with the Jews and Christians who were scattered throughout the Arabian Peninsula.

Two popular gods not represented by idols in the Kaaba were Shams (the goddess of sun), and Lah, god of the moon. When the prefix "al" (similar to the word "the" in English) is combined with "Lah," the result is "Allah," the full name of this ancient moon god. Allah's association with the moon is the reason why a crescent is often seen on flags and mosques of Islamic countries. If, in fact, Muhammad did worship Allah prior to becoming a prophet, he was certainly not the first to do so. But he was to become the first to extol Allah as the one and only god (Armstrong 1992).

As mentioned earlier, our knowledge of Muhammad's childhood is limited; however, the information collected in this chapter clearly demonstrates the difficulties that Muhammad faced since early childhood. Also, there is a clear indication that his troubled childhood did not lead him to psychopathy. Rather, he became pious with a strong sense of right and wrong. In a society in which wars and killings were everyday occurrences, Muhammad grew up to be honest and conservative. He was careful with everything he said and he did. His obsession with religion and his compulsive ritualistic behaviors led him to the next phase of his tumultuous life.

CHAPTER 3

THE FIRST REVELATIONS

اقْرَأ بِاسْمِ رَبِّكَ الَّذِي خَلَقَ

Read in the name of your Lord who created.
—The *Quran*, 96:1

In order to fully explore the life of Muhammad, it is important to first understand the *Quran* and the Hadith. *Quran* is an Arabic word meaning "to recite." It is the written account of Muhammad's divine revelations, collected in one book. Hadith is an Arabic word meaning "an event or a story." Over the course of time, the word has come to mean "quotations or stories related to the prophet Muhammad." The religion of Islam is therefore built on the *Quran* and the Hadith—what Muhammad claimed to have received from God and what he did during the course of his life.

THE QURAN

The *Quran* is different from the books of other religions. There is only one version of the *Quran,* and most Islamic scholars promote learning and reading it in its original language to prevent misinterpretations. All Moslems in the world recite the same book. Muhammad himself is said to have loved the *Quran* and was always pleased to hear it being recited.

The *Quran* is divided into 114 sections called *suras*. Some of these *suras* are long and some contain just a few lines. Each *sura* is divided into several verses, or *ayahs*. The verses of the *Quran* are mostly small and are made up of a few words, although some of them are much longer. Short or long, most of the verses are rhythmic and rhyme in several dimensions. The quality of these sentences in Arabic are quite superior to what most other writers have produced throughout the centuries.

The Hadith

If someone reports that there is a Hadith related to an issue, this usually means that there is a documented story somewhere regarding what Muhammad said or did on that particular topic. During the last years of Muhammad's life, the people around him recognized that they were witnessing history. Many of these people told and retold accounts of Muhammad's teachings. Although there is only one version of the *Quran*, there are multiple books written regarding Hadith, and most of these are accepted as valuable stories. Most of the books on the Hadith contain the interpretation of the Hadith based on the author's Islamic sect and his personal beliefs. In total contrast to the *Quran*, the Hadith has numerous variations and has been exploited by many people to achieve their ambitions.

Another problem with these stories of Hadith is that many were written after Muhammad's death. In fact, the number of stories increased dramatically over time. By the time Muhammad had been dead for 150 years, the collections of Hadith stories had grown to more than 250,000. To address this problem, Muhammad's biographers decided to take on the task of separating the credible stories from those that were clearly fabricated. The work of these biographers is now the main source of knowledge regarding Muhammad's life.

Many of these biographers spent their lifetime traveling the Islamic empire gathering stories, sayings, quotes, and teachings related to Mohammed and then painstakingly recreating Muhammad's life based

The First Revelations

on these Hadith. Some of these books are incredibly detailed and give a reasonably accurate account of Muhammad's life and character. While these authors' styles of reporting are dissimilar to the modern form used in scientific journals, there is no doubt that they were honest and knew what they were doing.

As Muhammad's biographers dug through the masses of stories, they encountered many problems. There was one subject, however, on which there was much agreement: the Hadith regarding Muhammad's famous first encounter with angel Gabriel. This story is mostly derived from report of Muhammad's wife Aysha. Aysha was Muhammad's favorite wife; she knew the *Quran* by heart and was to become an important figure in history and politics of Islam after Muhammad's death. Since Aysha was not around at the time of these events, she most likely heard the story from Muhammad himself.

THE FIRST CONTACT

As Muhammad's life unfolds, odd habits and behaviors begin to surface. For instance, Muhammad began spending long periods of time in the caves outside of Mecca in order to get away from the crowds in the city. It is not known whether this was a common practice at the time—in more recent times, this type of withdrawal from society to worship in the mountains is not commonly practiced in the Middle East. Certainly, if privacy was the goal, Muhammad could have found this within his own house.

Muhammad's withdrawal to the caves raised eyebrows among his neighbors. After spending time visiting the cave, Muhammad would return to walk around the Kaaba and indulge in various religious rituals. It is clear from his behavior that he was preoccupied with religious matters and was probably trying to come to grips with some existential issues. The concept of atonement through sacrifice and self-deprivation was common and was believed to lead to a higher level of consciousness among practitioners.

Most authors have concluded that Muhammad was probably seeking atonement and was spending his time in the mountains in prayer and meditation. Whatever the case, some major changes took place in Muhammad during this time. In particular, it is reported that he began having true dreams.

> Muhammad Ibnu Umar reported . . . he heard Aysha say: "The first things ever to be revealed to the Apostle of Allah (PBUH) were his night dreams that came to be true. He never dreamt of anything that did not happen afterwards just like a break of dawn. He remained so for quite a while. He liked solitude like nothing else and used to go into retreat in the cave of Hira for nights before returning home to Khadijeh. That prevailed until revelation caught him off-guard while he was in the cave. (Ibn Saad, Arabic, reprinted 1990, 1:153)

Muhammad made a practice of spending part of the holy month of Ramadan in the cave of Hira just outside Mecca. During his stay, which sometimes lasted for many days, he would give food to the poor in the area and spend much time in prayer. When he returned to Mecca, Muhammad would do his ritualistic walk around the Kaaba before going home.

On one particular night during the sacred month of Ramadan, most likely the month of June of 610 C.E (Mostofi 1998, 135) Muhammad was meditating alone in his cave when the archangel Gabriel appeared to him. The angel commanded him to read; to which the illiterate Muhammad replied, "I cannot read." The angel then squeezed Muhammad as if to draw the very life from his body and again commanded him to read. Once again, the frightened Muhammad replied that he could not, after which the angel squeezed Muhammad to within an inch of his life and ordered him once more to read. At that moment, it is said the first *sura* was revealed to Muhammad (Al-Bukhari 1988, 1:5)

Muhammad's Self-Doubt

The Prophet would later report that the encounter with the angel was forever written on his heart. This famous first *sura*, (number 96 in current Quran), is quite poetic and is a delight to read in Arabic.

اقْرَأْ بِاسْمِ رَبِّكَ الَّذِي خَلَقَ

Read in the name of your Lord Who created.

خَلَقَ الْإِنْسَانَ مِنْ عَلَقٍ

He created man from a clot of congealed blood:

اقْرَأْ وَرَبُّكَ الْأَكْرَمُ

Read and your Lord is most Honorable,

الَّذِي عَلَّمَ بِالْقَلَمِ

Who taught (to write) with the pen.

عَلَّمَ الْإِنْسَانَ مَا لَمْ يَعْلَمْ

Taught man what he knew not.

Most historians interpret this section to mean that God was assuring Muhammad that he did not need to fear his illiteracy. He who was able to create man from "a clot of congealed blood" and create the human capacity to read and write would be merciful to Muhammad and make certain that he, too, would be able to read (Ayatollah Makarem Shirazi 1995, 27:158).

When the angel left him, Muhammad was frightened and confused. Unable to make sense of the encounter, Muhammad worried that he had become possessed by demons or had grown delusional. He was so upset by the incident that he even contemplated suicide by throwing himself off the mountain. But another vision stopped him. Muhammad saw the angel again, this time seated on a throne on the horizon. The angel told

Muhammad that he was the archangel Gabriel and that he had been sent to relay messages to Muhammad from God. Muhammad, the angel said, had been chosen to be a prophet. When Muhammad looked around, he saw that the angel was surrounding him all directions.

Meanwhile, back in Mecca, Muhammad's wife, Khadijeh, had become worried that he had not yet come home, so she sent someone to find him. Eventually, a terrified Muhammad returned on his own, only to take to his bed, hide under a blanket, and beg Khadijeh to keep him covered. As he related the events of the day to his concerned wife, Muhammad confessed his fear that he had somehow become a sorcerer or gone mad. Khadijeh consoled Muhammad and tried to reassure him that he had not lost his sanity. She reasoned that Muhammad's piousness and innate goodness would surely prevent Allah from doing him any harm (Ibn Saad 1990, 1:152–153).

Khadijeh had an uncle who had read the Bible and was familiar with stories of the biblical prophets. This uncle had converted to Christianity. Khadijeh and Muhammad decided to visit him in the desert where he lived. Upon hearing their story, the uncle assured them that Muhammad was undoubtedly a true prophet and was not suffering from delusions. But the uncle also issued an ominous warning: People singled out in this way by God were likely to face a great deal of hardship. He predicted that Muhammad's own people would reject him and that his life as a prophet would be difficult. While Muhammad was glad to hear that he was not crazy, his encounter with Khadijah's uncle still did not remove every shadow of doubt about his sanity and his mission from his mind.

It took nearly three years for Muhammad to finally accept and embrace his mission and publicly announce his new-found religion. Even then, some believe that he continued to face grave self-doubts. (It should be noted that not every Islamic theologian believes that Muhammad faced self-doubt. However, there are many Hadith and verses of the *Quran* that indicate Muhammad was, in fact, less than confident in the early years of Islam.)

The First Revelations

مَا أَنتَ بِنِعْمَةِ رَبِّكَ بِمَجْنُونٍ

By the grace of your Lord you are not mad. (68:2)

The following Hadith is a famous story from the book of *Suhaily*. It refers to Muhammad's questioning of his unusual experience and of Khadijah's efforts to help him make sense of his first encounter with the angel Gabriel.

Khadijeh said to the prophet, "Oh cousin, could you let me know when your friend, the one who comes to you, when he comes?" He said yes. She said, "So if he comes, let me know." Then Gabriel PBUH (Peace Be Upon Him) came to him as he used to do. So the prophet said to Khadijeh, "Oh Khadijeh, this is Gabriel; he has come to me." She said, "Get up cousin and sit on my left leg." So the prophet got up and sat on her leg. She said, "Do you see him?" He said, "Yes." She said, "Move over and sit on my right leg." And the prophet moved over and sat on her right leg. She said, "Do you see him?" He said, "Yes, "So she said, "Move over and sit on my lap." So the prophet moved over and sat on her lap. She said, "Do you see him?" He said, "Yes." So she removed her veil and set it aside while the prophet was sitting on her lap, then said. "Do you see him?" He said, "No". She said, "Cousin, remain and rejoice, for, by God, this is no devil. This is an angel." (Suhaily, Arabic, reprinted 1977, 157)

At some point during these early experiences, there was a period of time when Muhammad's revelations abruptly stopped. Muhammad, clearly confused by this turn of events, worried that God had forsaken him. Some historians report that by this time, others in Mecca knew of Muhammad's ordeal and had begun to publicly ridicule him. As this ridicule increased, Muhammad became more and more frightened and confused (Ibn Ishaq, 155). It is not known how long this period lasted—

it may have been as short as a couple of days or as long as several weeks. In any case, it ended as suddenly as it had begun and the visions came flooding back. The revelations continued until Muhammad's death.

The following *sura*, "Almodather," is believed to be the second *Sura* of the *Quran*. In this *sura*, Muhammad is told to stop worrying that God has abandoned him and to get up and carry on with his mission.

يَا أَيُّهَا الْمُدَّثِّرُ

O you who are clothed!

قُمْ فَأَنذِرْ

Arise and warn. (74:1–2)

Some historians believe that the first *sura* after the episode of silence was "Alduha," which is also among the more lyric sections of the *Quran*. An examination of the content of this *sura*, number 93, makes a convincing case for this claim.

مَا وَدَّعَكَ رَبُّكَ وَمَا قَلَى

Your Lord has not forsaken you, nor has He become displeased,

وَلَلْآخِرَةُ خَيْرٌ لَكَ مِنَ الْأُولَى

And surely what comes after is better for you than that which has gone before.

وَلَسَوْفَ يُعْطِيكَ رَبُّكَ فَتَرْضَى

And soon will your Lord give you so that you shall be well pleased.

أَلَمْ يَجِدْكَ يَتِيمًا فَآوَى

Did He not find you an orphan and give you shelter?

THE FIRST REVELATIONS

وَوَجَدَكَ ضَالًّا فَهَدَى

And find you lost (that is, unrecognized by men) and guide (them to you)?

وَوَجَدَكَ عَائِلًا فَأَغْنَى

And find you in want and make you to be free from want?

THE MIRACLE OF THE QURAN

When Muhammad's *Quran* was introduced to the people of Arabia, it was met with great skepticism. Many argued that true prophets performed miracles and pointed to Jesus and Moses as examples. Where were Muhammad's miracles? Many reasoned that only those who could perform feats impossible for ordinary human beings could possibly prove that they were working under divine direction and inspiration. After all, when Moses' staff had become a writhing snake in front of a crowd of onlookers, it was easy to accept that he was not an average shepherd. Jesus could cure incurable diseases like leprosy and seizures and could bring the dead back to life, which was not a talent that every Jewish man could claim.

To convince his skeptics, Muhammad literally needed a miracle. His miracle, he said, was the fact that he had been transformed overnight from an illiterate merchant into a gifted linguist, and that the *Quran* was his miracle. Muhammad maintained this claim as the sole miracle of his ministry throughout his life.

Muhammad soon began the early stages of attempting to recruit converts to Islam. He began with those closest to him: his wife Khadijeh and his cousin Ali, who was just 10 years old at the time. Muhammad introduced himself as a prophet and "the messenger of Allah" and invited them to follow him, which they did. Khadijeh and Ali became the very first Muslims (Ibn Ishaq, P111–114).

The Intellect of Muhammad

Muhammad's life is unique in many respects. Many factors had to come together for him to accomplish all that he did. Like other significant events in history, minor events could have altered his path in life. His ability to come up with the *Quran* is not unique in itself.

There are those who believe that the *Quran* is far from perfect and that other Arab writers have matched its quality. These critics claim to have found grammatical errors and other flaws in the *Quran* and contend that though it is a fine piece of literature, it is by no means unique, and, by extension, neither is its author (Dashti [Persian], 229–269). However, the purpose of this book is not to conduct a comparative literary study but to report the accepted historical fact that the *Quran* is regarded as extremely high quality Arabic literature, if not the best ever written.

Even when accepting the fact that the *Quran* is exceptionally fine literature, the question still remains: How could such a work have been created so suddenly by a man known to have been illiterate? The answer is simply Muhammad's extremely high intelligence, which is seen in his life from the day in the cave of Hira until his death.

We can detect Muhammad's intellect in many aspects of his life. In the span of just 23 years, his influence effectively transformed a backward tribal society into a force capable of conquering most of the world known to Arabs of the time. Historically, those who have had such a major impact on their respective societies were highly intelligent individuals. There is much evidence to support the notion that Muhammad had a high IQ. His eloquence, tolerance, and abilities to persuade, negotiate, foresee possible outcomes, and make wise decisions all point to his superior intellect

The Unique Qualities of the Quran

The *Quran* is clearly an impressive piece of literature, but in many ways it is inherently different from other Arabic writings of the time. There are about 10 major types of Arabic poetry that are differentiated from one another by their method of rhyme. Writers skilled in the art of rhyme were hailed as talented poets. But the *Quran* did not fit into any existing Arabic poetic or literary category. It was written, instead, in the tradition of the Bible, with a complex mix of long and short verses. These verses showed a sophistication of rhyme that was so magnificent many believed it must have been divinely inspired. Muhammad often challenged his critics to compose even one line that was equivalent in beauty to any in the *Quran*. No one met the challenge.

Muhammad was able to transform his ideas into the shape of biblical writings that were so pleasant and beautiful that few readers could resist them. These writings were also rich in multidimensional rhymes, which explain why 1,500 years after the *Quran* was first written it still inspires awe. Authors who try to debunk Muhammad by devaluing his writings make a grave error. Whatever one may think of Muhammad, his ability to transfer profound thoughts into writing was exceptional, especially in light of the fact that he was an illiterate, small-time merchant. It is easy to see why many, both then and now, consider the *Quran* a miracle.

Although the *Quran* is a magnificent piece of Arabic literature, a look through world literature demonstrates that most languages can boast at least one writer whose talent was so great that it has never been duplicated. Most literary scholars agree that Shakespeare was one such example—his writing is widely acknowledged as the best of its kind in the English language. Of course, Shakespeare and Muhammad cannot really be compared side by side. The two were from vastly different backgrounds, and the impetus for their writings was also vastly different. While Shakespeare wrote for his own reasons, Muhammad wrote to express God's revelations to his Arab countrymen. However, although the purpose of the writing may have been different, the quality of the works produced by both men is exceptional and hard to match.

ALEF LAM MIM

Some of the *suras* begin with a verse that is made up of a few disconnected Arabic letters that have no real meaning. For example, several begin with the letters *A-L-M* while another starts with *A-L-M-S*. When Muhammad was asked about the meaning of these disconnected letters (referred to as *Alef-Lam-Mim*), he would only reply, "I do not know, these are secrets of the *Quran*, and God is the only one who knows it."

During recent years, there has been an attempt to count the number of different words in the *Quran*. This practice is similar to what many people have tried to do with the Bible—deciphering its secrets by turning it into numbers. But a look at these *suras* in the *Quran* quickly reveals the origin of these mysterious letters—it appears that the investigators were focusing on the trees so much that they could not see the forest. For example, the first verse of *sura* 38 is the single letter *saad*, the Arabic equivalent of the letter *S*. The letter *S* occurs more frequently in this *sura* than other sections of the *Quran*. The first verse of *sura* 68 is the single letter *noon*, the Arabic equivalent of the letter *N* in English. *Sura* 68 contains a higher percentage of the letter *N* than other parts of the *Quran*. The same rule applies to *sura* 50 that refers to the letter *Ghaf*, the equivalent of *gh* in English.

The rule continues to apply to some of the longer *suras* that were written over a longer period of time, but the difference is not as pronounced and requires more complex mathematics to elicit actual percentages, which probably explains why our predecessors did not notice the differences. As mentioned earlier, the *Quran*, similar to other good literature, rhymes in several dimensions. The use of certain letters in a given *sura* would add to the beauty of that section and probably was one of the elements that Muhammad had in mind while creating his book

Muhammad's Defense of the Quran

The real question is not whether or not Muhammad was truly a poet, but rather: Why would an intelligent, upstanding citizen like Muhammad suddenly decide that he was a prophet of God on a divine mission to lead the world toward a new religion? And why would he do it knowing full well the cost that he, his family, and his clan would have to pay?

THE FIRST REVELATIONS

Were his revelations truly sent from God? If not, what was happening in his mind that caused him to believe they were? And finally, why did Muhammad leave a simple but secure life for a journey of a thousand problems?

When Muhammad's work was first distributed in Mecca, many dismissed it as satanic and evil poetry. Muhammad's response to these criticisms is recorded in what is known as the section of poets in the *Quran*, the "Shoara."

هَلْ أُنَبِّئُكُمْ عَلَى مَن تَنَزَّلُ الشَّيَاطِينُ

Shall I inform you (of him) upon whom the Shaitans descend?

تَنَزَّلُ عَلَى كُلِّ أَفَّاكٍ أَثِيمٍ

They descend upon every lying, sinful one,

يُلْقُونَ السَّمْعَ وَأَكْثَرُهُمْ كَاذِبُونَ

They incline their ears, and most of them are liars.

وَالشُّعَرَاءُ يَتَّبِعُهُمُ الْغَاوُونَ

And as to the poets, those who go astray follow them.

أَلَمْ تَرَ أَنَّهُمْ فِي كُلِّ وَادٍ يَهِيمُونَ

Do you not see that they wander about bewildered in every valley?

وَأَنَّهُمْ يَقُولُونَ مَا لَا يَفْعَلُونَ

And that they say that, which they do not do.

إِلَّا الَّذِينَ آمَنُوا وَعَمِلُوا الصَّالِحَاتِ وَذَكَرُوا اللَّهَ كَثِيرًا وَانتَصَرُوا مِن بَعْدِ مَا ظُلِمُوا وَسَيَعْلَمُ الَّذِينَ ظَلَمُوا أَيَّ مُنقَلَبٍ يَنقَلِبُونَ

Except those who believe and do good and remember Allah much, and defend themselves after they are oppressed; and they who act unjustly shall know to what final place of turning they shall turn back. (26:221–227)

In other words, Muhammad was saying, "Do you want me to tell you who are the people who dispense satanic poetry? They are liars and sinners. The purpose of Satan is to be bad, to destroy, to be sneaky, to corrupt, and to try to create derelicts and destruction. People who like him are the sinners and liars. None of these apply to the *Quran*. So Muhammad cannot be from Satan. So the *Quran* cannot be the rule of Satan." (Ayatollah Makarem Shirazi 1995, 15:374–377).

Most of the *Quran* focuses on monotheism, truth, justice, and reform in all aspects of life—not exactly the kind of subjects likely to have been inspired by Satan. But Muhammad's critics did not stop at challenging the *Quran*. Muhammad was accused by some of being delusional and was referred to as *majanoon*, or the "psychotic poet." The *ayah* 36 of the *sura* "Safat" refers to this issue:

وَيَقُولُونَ أَئِنَّا لَتَارِكُوا آلِهَتِنَا لِشَاعِرٍ مَّجْنُونٍ

And to say: What! Shall we indeed give up our gods for the sake of a mad poet? (37:36)

This verse clearly suggests that Muhammad's pagan critics were struggling with the notion that they were being asked to abandon their own gods to follow the "crazy poet." But the *Quran* offers a defense of Muhammad's character, pointing out that most poets were people of low stature who were continuously after women, wine, and gold. Such poets used their art to vent their emotions and to woo the opposite sex. Other poets wrote grand poems glorifying the tribal leaders, for which they were paid handsomely. The writings of the *Quran*, however, were focused solely on teaching an ideology. In contrast to those poets whose works often focused on human pleasures, the *Quran* primarily taught self-control and morality. Other poets wrote for money, power, notoriety, or sex. But Muhammad wrote to teach. The *Quran* taught that God was omnipotent and more powerful and trustworthy than idols carved of wood or stone. It called readers to curtail their evil behaviors and to put their trust in a higher power.

Muhammad had poets among his followers who used their craft to help further the cause of Islam. Muhammad sometimes used these poets' services in public negotiations. It was common when opposing sides were discussing a deal to go head-to-head in a sort of battle of words. Each side would prepare and deliver an eloquent speech detailing its point of view. Each side would then produce a poet to compose a few lines on their behalf. The side that offered the best speech and poem won the debate. When they were needed, Muhammad's poets would fulfill this role. Muhammad himself never got involved in the "business" of poetry, even when it was necessary (Ayatollah Makarem Shirazi 1995, 15:380).

CHAPTER 4

MUHAMMAD'S CONDITION

"ما أَحْبَبْتُ مِنْ عَيْشِ الدُّنْيَا إلا الطيب والنِّساء"

I have loved nothing in this life save for scent and women.

MUHAMMAD

It is commonly accepted in the medical community that subjects with higher than average IQs are more difficult to diagnose than patients of average intelligence. The challenge becomes even greater when the person in question does not live what could be termed a "normal life" within his culture. In other words, the less eventful and more ordinary the person's life is, the easier it will be to establish a diagnosis for that individual. This makes the diagnosis of Muhammad—an intelligent man whose life was far beyond ordinary—inherently more challenging. However, the evidence that Muhammad was indeed suffering from complex partial seizures is overwhelming.

DISTINCTIONS IN MUHAMMAD'S CONDITION

Early in his career, Muhammad's contemporaries called him *majanoon* (a term most likely used to refer to schizophrenics or other severely mentally-disabled individuals, equivalent to "crazy" in contemporary Arabic). This is not surprising—Muhammad admitted to having discussions with an angel on a regular basis, and his visual and auditory hallucinations must have made him seem quite *majanoon* indeed. Ancient Arabs had experience with *majanoons*. Studies have indicated that schizophrenia affects about one percent of every population, regardless of culture. Undoubtedly, there were schizophrenics in ancient Arabia, and it would not be surprising if many assumed Muhammad to be one.

However, there are important distinctions to be made in Muhammad's case; distinctions that Muhammad's contemporaries eventually came to realize. Schizophrenics tend to be scattered in their thoughts and lack focus. They also tend not to have the ego strength to make great achievements in life. It can be an ordeal just to get a schizophrenic patient to take his medicine regularly, let alone accomplish the achievements that Muhammad did as a man and as a leader of his people.

As an aside, I have studied schizophrenics in the United States and Iran, and I can confirm that, regardless of their location or culture, these patients tend to exhibit a universal set of personality traits and characteristics. Even their responses to tests such as the Rorschach are quite similar. In other words, the symptoms of schizophrenia are the same; the environmental factors only shape the expression of those symptoms. It is unlikely that the schizophrenics of ancient Arabia were terribly different from other schizophrenics in other countries or other times. Muhammad simply does not fit the profile of a schizophrenic then or now.

Over time, this fact became evident to those who were around Muhammad. He did not act like a crazy person. What set Muhammad apart even in the minds of those who wished to believe that he was "crazy" was his dedication to his beliefs, his ability to attract and captivate devotees, his skill in forming and carrying out elaborate plans, and his aptitude at forging contracts. Even after Muhammad and his entire clan were banished from Mecca and forced to live outside the city in desperate poverty, Muhammad remained a forceful leader and managed to maintain the loyalty of his followers. In a society in which war played a major role, later on, Muhammad and his band claimed one victory after another. Schizophrenic patients simply do not possess this kind of high-level of functioning and long-term vision.

In addition, despite the fact that Muhammad was continually accused of being crazy or having been overtaken by demons, there is no indication that he was ever accused of having seizures. Seizure disorders were relatively common in Muhammad's day, and his countrymen had certainly been exposed to the phenomenon. It thus seems strange that someone would not have noted these seizures if Muhammad had indeed suffered from them.

This is especially unusual given the fact that Muhammad's enemies often sought for tools to use against him, as the following story shows:

> When the fair was due, a number of the Ghouraish came to Al-Walled b. al-Mughira, who was a man of some standing, and he addressed them in these words: "The time of the fair has come around again and representatives of the Arabs will come to you and they will have heard about this fellow of yours, so agree upon one opinion without dispute so that none will give the lie to the other." They replied, "You give us your opinion about him." He said, "No, you speak and I will listen." They said, "He is a kahin [at the time, this was a type of charlatan clergyman or fortuneteller]. He said, "By God, he is not that, for he has not the unintelligent murmuring and rhymed speech of the kahin." "Then he is possessed," they said. "No, he is not that," he said, "we have seen possessed ones and here are no choking, spasmodic movements and whispering." "Then he is a poet," they said. "No, he is no poet, for we know poetry in all its forms and meters." "Then he is a sorcerer." "No, we have seen sorcerers and their sorcery, and there is no spitting and no

knots." "Then what are we to say, O Abu 'Abdu Shams?" they asked. He replied, "By God, his speech is sweet, his root is a palm-tree whose branches are fruitful and everything you have said would be known to be false. The nearest thing to the truth is your saying that he is a sorcerer, who has brought a message by which he separates a man from his father, or from his brother, or from his wife, or from his family." (Ibn Ishaq, P 121)

Had any of Muhammad's contemporaries observed what they believed to be an overt sign of seizures, they would surely have used that information to discredit Muhammad's visions and his life's mission. The cause of this confusion then, and indeed through out the centuries, has been the fact that Muhammad did not suffer from grand mall seizures, and his symptoms were much more subtle and thus more likely to be overlooked by those around him. He did not fall violently and did not exhibit any of the other common symptoms of grand mal seizures, such as foaming at the mouth.

A careful study of Muhammad's condition shows that he suffered from complex partial seizures, which are difficult to observe and do not cause the obvious symptoms of a typical seizure. Although history shows us that Muhammad's symptoms did become more severe and overt as he aged, by that time, he had developed a devoted following who explained away his symptoms as being caused by the pressure of communing with angels. It is interesting to note that when people around Muhammad saw the epileptic attack, they—along with Muhammad—assumed that it was the pressure of the divine experience.

Muhammad's Symptoms

People suffering from temporal lobe epilepsy (complex partial seizures) usually display several distinct symptoms: olfactory hallucinations, epigastric sensation, auditory hallucinations and visual hallucinations, as well as excessive perspiration, among other problems. (please refer to appendix I for the details)

Olfactory Hallucinations

Olfactory hallucinations normally manifest as unpleasant smells. These types of hallucinations occur when changes in the brain during a seizure cause the patient to experience an unpleasant smell that does not have an external cause. During the nineteenth century, such seizures were referred to as "uncinate fits"—a reference to the olfactory center in the brain, which controls smell (Moore 1997).

Victims of olfactory hallucinations may suffer from a bad smell both before and after the seizure. As a result, many patients with complex partial seizures become hypersensitive to odors and spend their lives trying to avoid bad smells or cover them up with perfumes and colognes. Muhammad displayed this kind of sensitivity to unpleasant odors. When he was asked what pleasures he preferred among all those in life, he had two answers—women and perfume.

أخبرنا موسى بن إسماعيل، أخبرنا أبو بشر صاحب البصري عن يونس عن الحسن

قال: قال رسول الله، صلعم،: "ما أحْبَبْتُ مِنْ عَيْشِ الدّنْيَا إلا الطيب والنّساء"

Mussa Ibnu Ismail reported that . . . Al Hassan heard the Apostle of Allah (PBUH) say: "I have loved nothing in this life save for scent and women." (Ibn Saad 1990: 1:304)

Although Muhammad was by nature a generous person and was careful when it came to accepting gifts, he never said no when presented with fragrance.

أخبرنا الفضل بن دكين، أخبرنا عزرة بن ثابت، حدّثني ثمامة بن عبد الله بن أنس أن

أنسا كان لا يردَ الطيب، وزعم أن رسول الله، صلعم، كان لا يردَ الطيب

Ibnu Dukein narrated that . . . Abdullah Ibnu Anas said that Anas never refused when offered scent, and said that the Apostle of Allah (PBUH) also never did (Ibn Saad 1990, 1:305).

As much as he hated bad smells, Muhammad was quite fond of pleasant ones and often wore perfume. Those who knew him could "smell him coming" so to speak, because of his heavy scent.

أخبرنا موسى بن إسماعيل ابو سلمة، أخبرنا أبو بشر صاحب البصري، أخبرنا يزيد الرقاشي أن أنس بن مالك قال: كنا نعرف خروج النبيّ، صلعم، بريح الطيب.

Mussa Ibnu Ismail Abu Salma related . . . Anas Ibnu Malik said: "We used to know the Apostle of Allah was coming out by the fragrance of the scent he used to wear." (Ibn Saad 1990, 1:305)

Muhammad even had a favorite scent:

أخبرنا موسى بن إسماعيل، أخبرنا أبو بشر، أخبرنا عبد الله بن عطاء المكّي عن محمد بن علي قال قلت لعائشة، رضي الله عنها: يا أمّه أكان رسول الله، صلعم، يتطيّب؟ قالت: نعم بذكارة الطيب، قلت: وما ذكارة الطيب؟ قالت: المسك والعنبر

Mussa Ibnu Ismail related that . . . Muhammad Ibnu Ali said, "I said to Aysha, may Allah be pleased with her: 'O Woman, did the Apostle of Allah (PBUH) wear scent?' She said: 'Yes, he did. He used to wear the *Dikara* of all scent?' I said: 'What is Dikara?' She said: 'Musk and ambergris.'" (Ibn Saad 1990, 1:305)

There are also several Hadith indicating that Muhammad's least favorite foods were onions and garlic. He also did not like people with yellow teeth, as they probably had bad breath.

The Prophet said, "Whoever has eaten garlic or onion should keep away from us (or should keep away from our mosque)." (Al-Bukhari 1998, *7: bk. 65, n. 363*)

Epigastric Sensation

Another physiological symptom common in sufferers of complex partial seizures is epigastric sensation. Patients with complex partial seizures often endure strong feelings of nausea accompanied by a bitter taste. Oddly, the bad taste is usually confined to only one side of the tongue and mouth. Most patients report that the best fix for this unpleasant condition is to eat sweets. The stickiness of sugar tends to remain in the mouth for a time, bringing continued relief by camouflaging the bad taste. Frequent brushing of the teeth can also help.

Biographies of Muhammad frequently report that his favorite foods were sweets, especially honey and halva. Halva is a Middle Eastern treat made of honey, spices, and rose water (it is similar to baklava). It is sweet, sticky, and sweet smelling, eaten with bread and milk, halva can be a full meal.

أخبرنا أبو أسامة حمّاد بن أسامة، أخبرنا هشام بن عروة عن أبيه عن عائشة، رضي الله

عنها، قالت: كان رسول الله، صلعم، يعجبه الحلو العسل

> Abu Osama Hammad Ibnu Osama reported that . . . Aysha, May Allah is pleased with her, said: "The Apostle of Allah used to appreciate Halva and honey." (Ibn Saad 1990, 1:298)

There is a famous story that when Muhammad's wives wanted his attention, they served him honey. Likewise, if one wife wanted to discredit another in the Prophet's eyes, she would claim that the other wife's honey was tainted with *maghafir*, a bad-smelling tree dropping that ruins the taste of whatever it touches. This, apparently, got his attention.

It appears that as with today's patients, Muhammad dealt with the bad taste by vigorously brushing his teeth—a fact that is well documented. One Hadith relates the extent of this need:

أخبرنا عفان بن مسلم أو غيره عن همّام بن يحيَ عن عليَ بن زيد قال: حدَّثنا أمَ

محمّد عن عائشة، رضي الله عنها، أن النبيّ، صلعم، كان لا يرقدُ ليلا ولا نهارا فيستيقظ إلاَ

تسوَّك قبل أن يتوضأ

Affan Ibnu Muslim, reported that . . . Aysha, may Allah be pleased with her, said "each time the Prophet (PBUH) slept and awoke, whether it was night or day, he used siwak [the type of toothbrush used at the time, usually made of the soft branches of palm trees] before performing his ablutions." (Ibn Saad 1990, 1:374)

Apparently, Muhammad's practice of brushing his teeth was excessive and surprising to people around him. Muhammad did not know the true cause of the need, but that need was apparently so acute that it actually created problems with his gums:

أخبرنا موسى بن مسعود ابو حذيفة النهديَ البصريَ، أخبرنا عكرمة بن عمّار عن

شدَّاد بن عبد اللّه قال: كان السواك قد أحفى لثة رسول اللّه، صلعم

Mussa Ibnu Messud reported that . . . Sheddad Ibnu Abdullah says: "Siwak wore out the gums of the Prophet. (PBUH)" (Ibn Saad 1990, 1:375)

It is customary in most cultures to brush one's teeth late at night, but not common to do it several times during the night. However, it appears that Muhammad indulged in brushing his teeth during the night as well:

MUHAMMAD'S CONDITION

أخبرنا سعيد بن منصور، أخبرنا هُشَيْمْ قال: أخبرنا أبو حُرَة عن الحسن عن سعد بن هشام عن عائشة ان رسول الله، صلعم، كان يوضع له السواك من الليل، وكان استأنف السواك فكان إذا قام من الليل استاك، ثمَ توضأَ، ثمَ صلى ركعتين خفيفتين، ثمَ صلى ثماني ركعات، ثمَ أوتر

Said Ibnu Mansur reported that . . . Aysha said that the Prophet (PBUH) was provided siwak during nighttime, and whenever he woke up he used it, performed his ablutions, briefly prayed in two prostrations, then fully prayed in eight prostrations, and, finally, performed the Witr prayer. (Ibn Saad 1990, 1:375)

In Muhammad's case, there was a direct correlation between brushing his teeth and the nausea that is associated with gustatory symptoms of complex partial seizures, as the following Hadith clearly shows:

.أخبرنا عارم بن الفضل، أخبرنا حمّاد بن زيد بن غيلان بن جرير عن أبي هريرة عن أبيه قال: رأيت النبيَّ، صلعم، وهو يستّنَ بمسواك بيده، والمسواك في فيه، وهو يقول: "غاغا"، كأنه يتهوَّع.

Aarim Ibnu alFadhl reported that . . . Abu Hureira said he heard his father say: "I saw the Prophet (PBUH) hold a toothpick in his hand and one in his mouth while uttering 'Gha Gha,' as if he was on the verge of vomiting." (Ibn Saad 1990, 1:375)

Muhammad's gastric problems appear to have been so troublesome that he even broke the rules of fasting. His followers were surprised that the Prophet would ignore the prohibition on brushing teeth during a fast. But Muhammad was in constant need of brushing. He was known always to travel with his *siwak*.

أخبرنا الحجَّاج بن نصير، أخبرنا الحُسام بن مصَنّ عن قتادة عن عكرمة قال: استاك رسول اللّه، صلعم، بجريد رطب وهو صائم، فقيل لقتادة: إن أناساً يكرهونه، قال: استاك واللّه رسول اللّه، صلعم، بجريد رطب وهو صائم. أخبرنا الفضل بن دُكين قال: أخبرنا مندَل عن ثور عن خالد بن معْدان قال: كان رسول اللّه، صلعم، يسافر بالسواك.

"The Prophet (PBUH) cleaned his teeth with a tender palm tree stick while he was fasting," Qutada was told. But some people disapprove of teeth cleaning while fasting. Qutada replied, "By Allah, I saw the prophet clean his teeth with a tender palm tree stick while he was fasting . . . Whenever the Prophet (PBUH) went on a trip, he took siwak with him." (Ibn Saad 1990, 1:375)

On his death bed, Muhammad brushed his teeth more vigorously than usual—so much so as to capture the eyes of his followers who reported it (Ibn Saad 1990, 180). This event, along with other reports, suggests that Muhammad probably died of complications associated with seizure disorder.

Excessive Perspiring

A well-documented physiological symptom of complex partial seizures is sweating. Many people who experience a complex partial seizure sweat excessively, regardless of the temperature. There are many Hadith that make reference to this symptom in Muhammad. The most famous story is one in which Aysha relates having seen the Prophet sweating profusely at the time of a revelation.

"، قالت عائشة: ولقد رأيته ينزل عليه الوحي في اليوم الشديد البرد فيُفصم عنه وإنَّ جبينه ليتفصَّد عرقًا.

> I saw him during a revelation. It was on a freezing day; yet, when the revelation eased on him, sweat was running down his forehead. (Ibn Saad 1990, 155)

Other followers witnessed additional famous accounts of Muhammad's perspiration. In fact, many viewed Muhammad's excessive perspiring to be a sign that he was being inspirited, as the following Hadith relates:

> Somebody said, "O Allah's Apostle! Can the good bring forth evil?" The Prophet remained silent for a while. It was said to that person, "What is wrong with you? You are talking to the Prophet (PBUH) while he is not talking to you." Then we noticed that he was being inspired divinely. Then the Prophet wiped off his sweat and said, "Where is the questioner?" It seemed as if the Prophet liked his question. (Al-Bukhari 1988, *2: bk. 24, n. 544*)

Auditory and Visual Hallucinations

It is not difficult to find evidence in Muhammad's life of his auditory and visual hallucinations. In fact, one could argue that all of his face-to-face conversations with the angel Gabriel are evidence of such hallucinations. The following Hadith provides verification of these two types of hallucinations:

> Khadijeh said to the prophet, "Oh cousin, could you let me know when your friend, the one who comes to you, when he comes?" He said yes. She said, "So if he comes, let me know. Then Gabriel (PBUH) came to him as he used to do. So the prophet said to Khadijeh, "Oh Khadijeh, this is Gabriel; he has come to me." She said, "Get up cousin and sit on my left leg." So the prophet got up and sat on her leg. She said, "Do you see him?" He said, "Yes." She said, "Move over and sit on my

right leg." And the prophet moved over and sat on her right leg. She said, "Do you see him?" He said, "Yes, "So she said, "Move over and sit on my lap." So the prophet moved over and sat on her lap. She said, "Do you see him?" He said, "Yes." So she removed her veil and set it aside while the prophet was sitting on her lap, then said. "Do you see him?" He said, "No". She said, "Cousin, remain and rejoice, for, by God, this is no devil. This is an angel." (Suhaily, p. 157)

Many patients suffering from complex partial seizures have auditory and visual hallucinations in which they think they are hearing or seeing things, particularly the sound of a bell. Hearing the sound of a bell is one of the well known universal symptoms of complex partial seizure and one of the easiest to document. In biographies of the Prophet, there are many references to him telling other people that he heard the sound of a bell. Muhammad's description of this phenomenon speaks for itself:

أخبرنا حجين بن المثنى، أخبرنا عبد العزيز بن عبد الله بن أبي سلمة عن عمّه انه بلغه أنَ رسول اللّه، صلعم، كان يقول: "كان الوحْيْ يأتيني على نحْوَيْن: يأتيني به جبْريلْ فيُلقيه عليَ كما يُلقي الرَجُلْ على الرَجُلْ فذلك يتفلتْ مني ويأتيني في شيءٍ مثل الجرس حتَى يُخالط قلْبي فذاك لا يتفلتْ منّي".

Hudjein Ibnu Alumna reported that . . . His uncle was told that the Apostle of Allah (PBUH) used to say: "The revelation comes to me in two ways: From Gabriel just like a man to man conversing, and that escapes me; and with something like the ringing of a bell until it melts into my heart, and that I can grasp." (Ibn Saad 1990, 1:155)

OTHER SYMPTOMS

When Muhammad heard the bell (and at other times as well) he experienced some degree of shaking, which is a common occurrence in some cases of complex partial seizures. Because these seizures usually arise from the left temporal lobe, shaking is typically confined to the right side of the body. Shaking can range from mild to severe, but is sometimes absent altogether. In at least one Hadith, it is reported that Muhammad's shaking was severe enough to jolt the animal that he was riding:

أخبرنا محمد بن عمر الأسلمي، أخبرنا ابو بكر بن عبد الله بن أبي سبرة عن صالح بن محمد عن أبي سلمة بن عبد الرحمن عن أبي أروى الدوسي قال: رأيت الوحي ينزل على النبيَّ، صلعم، وإنّه على راحلته، فترغو وتفتل يديها حتى أظن أن ذراعها تنفصم، فربما بركت وربما قامت موتّدة يديها حتى يُسرَى عنه من ثقل الوحي، وإنّه ليتحدّر منه مثل الجمان

> Mohammad Ibnu Umar Alaslami reported . . . Abu Urwa Aldussi told him: "I witnessed a revelation to the Apostle of Allah (PBUH) while he was on his mount. The animal bellowed and twisted its legs until I felt they would break; this went on until the weight of the revelation eased; when it did, he was soaked through with sweat." (Ibn Saad 1990: 1:155)

There are few references to Muhammad having been prone to falls, but the story told in one Hadith is significant. In this particular Hadith, Muhammad was about age 35 when he suffered a fall and lost consciousness:

> Narrated Jaber bin Abdullah: When the Kaaba was rebuilt; the prophet (PBUH) and Abbas went to carry stones. Abbas said to the prophet, "[take off and] put your waist sheet over your neck so that the stones may hurt you." [But as soon as he took off his waist sheet] he fell unconscious on the ground with both his eyes towards the sky. When he came to his senses, he said "My waist sheet! My waist sheet" then he tied his waist sheet. (Al-Bukhari 1988, 5:108)

Another common symptom of complex partial seizures is known as the "grimace." As a result of the muscular changes during a seizure, victims tend to contort their faces. There are many Hadith that refer to Muhammad exhibiting such a face at the time of revelation, including the following:

أخبرنا عفان بن مسلم، أخبرنا حمّاد بن سلمة، أخبرنا قتادة عن الحسن عن حطان بن عبد الله الرقاشي عن غيادة بن الصامت أنّ النبيّ، صلعم، كان إذا نزل عليه الوحي كُرب له وتربّد وجهه

Affan Ibnu Muslim reported that . . . Uyada Ibnu Assamit said, "Whenever the Apostle of Allah (PBUH) was revealed something, he felt very afflicted and his face clouded." (Ibn Saad 1990, 1:154)

Ubeiduallah Ibnu Mussa Alabassi reported . . . Akruma said: "Whenever something was revealed to the Apostle of Allah (PBUH), he remained struck down for an hour of time as if he was drunk." (Ibn Saad 1990, 1:154)

Along with the grimace, there are also references to Muhammad making noises during the revelation, which is again consistent with the symptoms of complex partial seizure.

Narrated Safwan bin Yahia bin Umaya from his father, who said, "A man came to the prophet while he was at Jirana, the man was wearing a cloak which had traces of Khaluq or Sufra [a kind of perfume]. The man asked [the Prophet], what do you order me to perform in my Umra? So, Allah inspired the prophet divinely and he was screened by a piece of cloth. I wished to see the prophet being divinely inspired. Umar said to me, "Come. Will you be pleased to look at the prophet while Allah is inspiring him?" I replied in the affirmative. Umar lifted one corner of the cloth and I looked at the prophet, who was snoring. [The sub-narrator said that the snoring was like that of a camel.] When that was over, the prophet asked, "Where is the questioner who asked about Umra? Put off your cloak and wash away the traces of Khaluq from your body and clean the sufra [yellow color] and perfume in your Umra what you perfume in your hajj. (Al-Bukhari 1988, 3:10)

Diagnosis

There is ample evidence that all of these experiences were directly caused by complex partial seizures. When the seizure originates in the left hemisphere of the brain, it creates problems in the muscles of the right side of the body. The following Hadith is one of the most complete reports of the Prophet's symptoms and their manifestations:

أخبرنا هاشم بن القاسم، أخبرنا عبد الحميد بن بَهرام قال: حدّثني شهر، حدّثني عبد الله بن عباس قال: بينما رسول اللّة، صلعم، بفناء بيته بمكّة جالسا إذ مرّ به عثمان بن مظعون، فكشر على رسول الله، صلعم، فقال له رسول الله، صلعم، : "ألا تجلس؟" قال: بلى، فجلس رسول الله مُستَقبله، فبينما هو يُحدّثه إذ شخص رسول الله، صلعم، فنظر ساعة إلى السّماء، فأخذ يضع بصره حتى وضعه على يمينه في الأرض، فتحرّف رسول الله، صلعم، عن جليسه عثمان إلى حيث وضع بصره، فأخذ يَنغِض رأسه كأنه يستفقه ما يُقال له، وابن مظعون ينظر، فلمّا قضى حاجته واستفقه ما يُقال له، وشخص بصر رسول الله، صلعم، إلى السّماء كما شخص أول مرة، فاتّبعه بصره حتى توارى في السّماء، فاقبل على عثمان بجلسته الأولى، فقال عثمان: يا محمّد فيما كنتْ أجالسك و آتيك ما رأيتك تفعل كفعلك الغداة، قال: "وما رأيتَني فعلتُ؟" قال: رأيتُك شخصت بصرك في السّماء ثمّ وضعته على يمينك فتحرّفت إليه وتركتني، فأخذت تنغض رأسك كأنك مُستَفقهه شيئا يُقال لك؟ قال: "أوفطنتَ لذاك؟" قال عثمان: نعم. قال: فقال رسول الله، صلعم، : "أتاني رسول الله آنفا وأنت جالسٌ"، قلتُ: رسولُ الله؟ قال: "نعم"، قال: فما قال

Hashim Ibnu Alqaasim reported . . . Abdullah Ibnu Abbas said, "As the Apostle of Allah (PBUH) was sitting in the courtyard of his home in Mecca, Othman Ibnu Madhuun passed by and smiled at him. The Apostle of Allah (PBUH) said, "Will you have a seat with me?" "Certainly," said Othman and sat facing him. As they were conversing, the Apostle of Allah (PBUH) stared at the sky for a long time and slowly moved his eyes to a spot on the ground on his right-hand and, turning his back on Othman, he started nodding his head as if he understood something said to him. Then he kept staring once more at the sky as if he was following something until it vanished. He, then, resumed the conversation with Othman. Othman said, "Oh Muhammad, as we were conversing a while ago, I saw you do something that I have never seen you do before." He said, "And what did you see me do?" Othman replied: "I saw you stare at the sky and, then, move your eyes slowly to the ground on your right-hand, turn your back on me, and leave me on my own." He said, "Did you realize all that?" Othman answered, "Indeed." The Apostle of Allah (PBUH) said, "As you were sitting, a messenger of Allah came to me." I said, "A messenger of Allah?" He said, "Yes." I said, "What did he say to you?" He replied, "Allah commands justice, the doing of good, and liberality to kith and kin, and He forbids all shameful deeds, and injustice and rebellion: He instructs you, that ye may receive admonition." Othman concluded, "It was at that very moment that faith settled in my heart and I loved Muhammad." (Ibn Saad 1990, 1:.138)

Although this is only one Hadith, it reveals several of Muhammad's symptoms occurring simultaneously; including what Muhammad calls a "vision." The author's honest and detailed reporting of what he saw shows how attuned his followers were to his behavior. The most interesting part of this Hadith is the author's indication that Muhammad's eyes were moving to the right, a clear sign that the origin of the seizure was in the left hemisphere of his brain.

At this point, it is possible to support the hypothesis that Muhammad suffered from left temporal lobe epilepsy. Further evidence includes the fact that he moved his lips and then admitted that he saw and spoke to someone who was not there. Clearly, when Muhammad was talking about having a one on one conversation with Gabriel, he was experiencing a hallucination caused by left temporal lobe epilepsy. The content of the hallucination was purely religious. And the most important point is that Muhammad completely believed that his hallucination was reality. He was not afraid of these hallucinations, which is evident in their frequency.

Although the author of the above Hadith does not mention whether Muhammad fell down in the description of seeing the angel face to face, this fact has been noted in other Hadith. In addition, it is evident that at other times Muhammad felt as if he were dying and heard the sound of bells. Each of these reports support the idea that some of Muhammad's seizures were more complicated and perhaps included both sides of his brain, causing him to become totally incapacitated, sweat profusely, shake, make noises, and afterwards become quiet and in need of rest.

TREATING THE SYMPTOMS

Bloodletting is an old method of treating diseases that was practiced by the Greeks (Aretaeus, c. A.D. 200) as well as by people of the Middle East up until recent times. There are many records that indicate Muhammad was a fan of this primitive and dangerous remedy. Although bloodletting has nothing to do with complex partial seizures, Muhammad's reasoning for engaging in this practice was to alleviate chronic headaches:

أخبرنا عفان بن مسلم، أخبرنا عبد الوارث بن سعيد، أخبرنا عبد العزيز بن صهيب عن الحسن قال: كان رسول الله، صلعم، يحتجم اثنتين في الأخدعيْن وواحدة في الكاهل، وكان يأمر بالوتْر.

Affan Ibnu Muslim reported . . . *Alhassan* said: "The Apostle of Allah (PBUH) used to practice two bloodlettings in the lower back of his head [the occipital area] and one in the upper part of his back and used to recommend a single bloodletting." (Ibn Saad 1990, 1:374)

Muhammad practiced bloodletting for many reasons. Interestingly, one of those reasons was to ward off potential mental problems:

أخبرنا هاشم بن القاسم، أخبرنا ليث، يعني ابن سعد، عن الحجّاج بن عبد اللذه الحميْري عن بكير بن الأشجّ قال: بلغني أن الأقرع بن حابس دخل على النبيّ، صلعم، وهو يحتجم في القمْحدُوَة فقال: يا بن ابي كبشة لم احتجمت وسط رأسك؟ فقال رسول الله، صلعم، : "يا ابنَ حابس إنّ فيها شفاءً من وجع الرَأس والأضْراس والنّعاس والمرض وأشْكَ في الجنون ليْت يشْكَ".

I heard that Alaqraa Ibnu Habis went to the Apostle of Allah (PBUH) and found him practicing bloodletting in the prominent part of a bone [apophasis]. Alaqraa said to him, "Oh Ibnu Abi Kabsha, why have you practiced bloodletting in the middle of your head?" The Apostle of Allah (PBUH) replied, "Oh Ibnu Habis, it is a relief from headaches, toothaches, sleeplessness, and illnesses, of which might be insanity." (Ibn Saad 1990, 1:374)

The Prophet also had an obsession with cleanliness. This compulsion can be observed in many aspects of Muhammad's life; however, it manifests itself most in instances relating to his urination. In his own life, Muhammad practiced exceptionally good hygiene. One Hadith states that: "Whenever the Prophet went to answer the call of nature, I used to bring water with which he used to clean his private parts" (Al-Bukhari 1988, 1: bk. 4, n. 216).

Muhammad went even further. In another *Hadith, the Prophet proscribes the practice of cleanliness for everyone, stating that if anyone fails in this, he or she is committing a major sin:*

> Once the Prophet, while passing through one of the graveyards of Medina or Mecca, heard the voices of two persons who were being tortured in their graves. The Prophet said, "These two persons are being tortured for a major sin. . . . Indeed, one of them never saved himself from being soiled with his urine while the other used to go about with calumnies [making enemy between friends]." The Prophet then asked for a green leaf of a date palm tree, broke it into two pieces, and put one on each grave. On being asked why he had done so, he replied, "I hope that their torture might be lessened, till these get dried." (Al-Bukhari 1988, 1: bk. 4, n. 215)

Although each one of these symptoms within and by themselves do not mean much, taken together they provide enough evidence to support the presence of an underling neurological disorder. Of course, there is more to complex partial seizures than a few symptoms. In the following chapters, I will provide the necessary evidence to establish the interconnection between the symptoms of the disease and the creation of Islam.

CHAPTER 5

PERSONALITY CHANGES: HYPER-RELIGIOSITY AND SEXUAL BEHAVIORS

أَتاني جِبْريلْ بِقدْرٍ فأكلْتْ منْها فأعْطيتْ قوَة أرْبعين رجْلا في الجِماع :

Gabriel came to me with an earthen pot; I ate from it and was endowed with the sexual potency of 40 men.

—Muhammad

One of the characteristics of complex partial seizures is a substantial personality change in the individual. This change is so profound that it appears as a total—but gradual—transformation of the individual into a different person. As with all seizure sufferers, some of the symptoms of Muhammad's condition are vivid while others are more subtle. One must dig diligently and deeply into his life to make order of the puzzle, including examining the revelations, the *vahy*, which mark the beginning of his prophethood.

RELIGIOUS THOUGHTS AND IMAGERY

Muhammad's accounts of his frequent encounters with the angel Gabriel give us some important clues into the nature of his condition. When asked how he received these visions, Muhammad replied that they came to him in two ways. The first was as one man talking to another. This, he said, was not difficult to tolerate. However, the revelations sometimes descended in much more disturbing ways. At these times, Muhammad reported hearing the sound of a bell "until it melted into my heart" and feeling as though the life was coming out of him. He never went through this experience, he said, without feeling that he was about to die.

> Narrated Aysha: Al-Harith bin Hisham asked Allah's Apostle. "O Allah's Apostle! How is the divine inspiration revealed to you?" Allah's Apostle replied, "Sometimes it is [revealed] like the ringing of a bell; this form of inspiration is the hardest of all, and then this state passes after I have grasped what is inspired. Sometimes the Angel comes in the form of a man and talks to me, and I grasp whatever he says." (Al-Bukhari, 1: bk. 1, n. 2)

During these seizures, Muhammad would be seized by a series of religious thoughts and images, which he would later recount for his followers. It is not surprising that these images would dominate his thinking during seizure attacks, as he was completely preoccupied with such thoughts and with his own sense of mission. It is also not surprising that his first experiences with visions were so frightening that he doubted his sanity. They were so real to him that once the sense of doubt was gone in his own mind, he had no mercy on people who doubted him.

Muhammad was a person who was honest, pious, and respected in his community. Suddenly, he experienced strange attacks in which the life seemed to go out of him. This orphan, whose money and prestige came primarily from his wife, then suddenly finds his own sense of mission—he is being called to be a prophet. It is important to note that Muhammad belonged to the group of Hanaffiya, who rejected idols in their search for a single god. Muhammad's mind had been ruminating on these topics for years until he had completely internalized the idea. These religious thoughts, coupled with his own need for a sense of mission, make it clear why the content of his thoughts would be of a religious nature when his seizures began.

Personality Changes: Hyper-Religiosity and Sexual Behaviors

Sexual Behavior

Besides hyper-religiosity, Muhammad developed other new behaviors that are closely associated with complex partial seizures. One of the most notable was hypersexuality. Muhammad did not marry until he was 25 years old, which was much older than other men of his time (most men married by the age of 16, and it was not unusual for girls to marry before the age of 10). Apparently, Muhammad did not even have any sexual experience before marriage—he was reported to have been a virgin at the time of his marriage (Mostofi 1988, 135).

Muhammad's Preoccupation with Women

After Muhammad finally married his first wife, Khadijeh, he did not marry again until after she died, when he was 53 years old. We know little about Muhammad and Khadijah's sex life except that the couple produced eight children (Al-Tabari 1990, Persian translation, 4:1288). However, after Khadijah's death, everything changed for Muhammad. He married two women at the same time: Aysha, a child of just six or seven, and an older woman named Sudeh, who had been married before.

Presumably, since Muhammad could not have intercourse with Aysha until she was older, he wed Sudeh for the purposes of sex and household management. Yet Aysha reports that when she was just seven years old, Muhammad had sex with her when no one was home (Al-Tabari, Persian translation, 1990, 4:1292). Although some authors point to Muhammad's marriage with Aysha as a sign of his pedophilia, it is well known that it was not unusual for men of the time to take very young girls as wives. The term "pedophiliac" does not apply to him.

Aysha and Sudeh were the second and third in what would be a long line of wives. According to Al-Tabari, Muhammad wed 15 wives, took 13 of them into his house, kept 11 of them together, and had 9 wives at home at the time of his death (Al Tabari, Persian translation, 1990, 4:1288).

There are those who claim that these marriages were primarily politically motivated and designed to forge alliances with various groups. However, two of Muhammad's wives (a woman from Bani Mostalgh and another captured in the battle of Khyber) were chosen by Muhammad for their beauty alone. In the case of the captured woman, Muhammad had sex with her the same night he killed her Jewish husband of four years. Would a politically motivated marriage engender this kind of lustful behavior? It is not likely. However, in the context of hypersexuality associated with complex partial seizures, Muhammad's behavior makes complete sense.

This unusual sexual desire in a man who was close to 60 years old must have caused curiosity among his people. In response to this question, there are several Hadiths in which Muhammad attributed his unusual sexual potency to the food given to him by the angel Gabriel:

أخبرنا عبيد الله بن موسى عن أسامة بن زيد عن صفوان بن سُليم قال: قال رسول الله، صلعم، :

"آتاني جبْريلُ بقدْرٍ فأكلْتُ منْها فأعْطيتُ قوّةَ أرْبعين رجُلاً في الجماع

> Abdullah Ibnu Mussa reported that . . . Safwan Ibn Suleim said the Apostle of Allah (PBUH) said, "Jibril (Gabriel) came to me with an earthen pot; I ate from it and was endowed with the sexual potency of 40 men." (Ibn Saad 1990, 1:282)

An important point to note in this Hadith is that Muhammad admitted his increased potency occurred *after* his encounter with Gabriel, which translates to the onset of the seizures. And there is more than just his word for this—there is his life. Muhammad manifested no signs of hypersexuality until his older years. (It should be noted that in Arabic, the number "40" is often used to indicate "a great deal" rather than the actual number. Such symbolic numbers are used in the Arabic language even today.) Suffice it to say, Muhammad was highly potent. Obviously, Muhammad was happy about this attribute and wished it on his devout followers.

Personality Changes: Hyper-Religiosity and Sexual Behaviors

أخبرنا مالك بن إسماعيل أبو غسّان، أخبرنا إسرائيل عن ليث عن مجاهد قال: أعطيَ رسول الله، صلعم، بُضْع أربعين رجلا و أعطيَ كلَ رجل من أهل الجنة بُضْع ثمانين

> Malik Ibnu Ismail Abu Ghassan reported . . . that Leith heard Mudjahid say: "The Apostle of Allah (PBUH) is endowed with the sexual potency of 40 men, and each man of the people of paradise is endowed with that of 80 men." (Ibn Saad 1990, 1:282)

In order to make it easier to act on his frequent sexual urges, Muhammad constructed a home with doors that opened into each of his wives' homes. He is said to have slept with a different woman each night (some accounts claim that Muhammad had sex with all of his wives, one after the other, every night; however, these reports are by nature difficult to corroborate.) One of the wives apparently forfeited her turn forever because she was no longer attractive and was afraid that Muhammad would divorce her. Four of his wives became his favorites.

In order to get his wives to give in to his desires, Muhammad used old-style maligning, calling it their religious duty:

> Narrated Abu Hureira: Allah's Apostle said, "If a husband calls his wife to his bed [i.e., to have sexual relation] and she refuses him to sleep in anger, the angels will curse her till morning." (Al-Bukhari 1988, 4:302)

Sometimes, Muhammad's sexual appetites got him into trouble. During one episode when some of Muhammad's followers were in Ethiopia, the Ethiopian king wished to give the Prophet a gift. Having heard about his penchant for beautiful women, the king presented him with a lovely young Christian slave girl named Mariah (Mary). Because Mariah did not have the status to live in Muhammad's house, the Prophet found a home for her on the outskirts of Medina and presumably visited her often.

One day, upon finding her in his house, Muhammad could not resist the temptation and took Mariah to Sudeh's bed. When Sudeh arrived home and found Muhammad and Mariah in bed together in her bed, she was furious. Muhammad promised to put aside Mariah forever if only Sudeh would not tell the others, but Sudeh spread the word regardless. Muhammad eventually decided that he should not be forced to forgo a pleasure given to him, especially when God comes to his aid:

يا أَيُّها النَّبِيُّ لم تُحرِّمْ ما أَحلَّ اللَّهُ لك تَبْتغي مرْضاتَ أَزْواجك واللَّهُ غَفورٌ رَحيمٌ

O Prophet! Why do you forbid (yourself) that which Allah has made lawful for you; you seek to please your wives; and Allah is Forgiving, Merciful?

قَدْ فرضَ اللَّهُ لكُمْ تَحلَّة أَيْمانكُمْ واللَّهُ موْلاكُمْ وهو الْعليمُ الْحكيمُ

Allah indeed has sanctioned for you the expiation of your oaths and Allah is your Protector, and He is the Knowing the Wise.

وإذْ أسرَّ النَّبِيُّ إلى بعْض أَزْواجه حديثًا فلمَّا نبَّأَتْ به وأَظْهرهُ اللَّهُ عليْه عرَّفَ بعْضهُ وأَعْرض عن بعْض فلمَّا نبَّأها به قالتْ منْ أَنبأَك هذا قال نبَّأني الْعليمُ الْخبيرُ

And when the prophet secretly communicated a piece of information to one of his wives—but when she informed (others) of it, and Allah made him to know it, he made known part of it and avoided part; so when he informed her of it, she said: Who informed you of this? He said: The Knowing, the one Aware, informed me.

إن تتوبا إلى اللَّه فقدْ صغتْ قُلوبُكُما وإن تظاهرا عليْه فإنَّ اللَّه هو موْلاهُ وجبْريلُ وصالحُ الْمُؤْمنين والْملائكة بعْد ذلك ظهيرٌ

If you both turn to Allah, then indeed your hearts are already inclined (to this); and if you back up each other against him, then

PERSONALITY CHANGES: HYPER-RELIGIOSITY AND SEXUAL BEHAVIORS

surely Allah it is Who is his Guardian, and Gabriel and the believers that do good, and the angels after that are the aiders.

عسى ربُّه إن طلقكنَ أن يُبدله أزواجا خيرا منكنَ مسلمات مؤمنات قانتات تائبات عابدات سائحات ثيِّبات وأبكارا

Maybe, his Lord, if he divorces you, will give him in your place wives better than you, submissive, faithful, obedient, penitent, adorers, fasters, widows and virgins. (The *Quran*, 66:1–5)

MUHAMMAD'S JUSTIFICATION

Another example of Muhammad's preoccupation with women can be found in the rules he established regarding the taking of wives. Because of frequent wars and deaths of men, many women and children found themselves suddenly alone. It was therefore permissible for a man to take as many wives as he wished. But Muhammad disagreed with the concept of a limitless number of wives. Instead, he declared that his followers should have only four wives each (women obtained as booty in war were an exception—a man could have as many of these or as many slave women as he wished as long as he married only four of them). There was one notable exception to the rule: Muhammad himself. Why would the Prophet place himself above his own law? The *Quran* provides some explanation:

يا أيُّها النَّبي إنا أحللنا لك أزواجك اللاتي آتيت أجورهنَ وما ملكت يمينك ممَّا أفاء اللَّه عليك وبنات عمِّك وبنات عمَّاتك وبنات خالك وبنات خالاتك اللاتي هاجرن معك وامرأة مؤمنة إن وهبت نفسها للنَّبي إن أراد النَّبي أن يستنكحها خالصة لك من دون المؤمنين قد علمنا ما فرضنا عليهم في أزواجهم وما ملكت أيمانهم لكيلا يكون عليك حرج وكان اللَّه غفورا رحيما

O Prophet! Surely We have made lawful to you your wives whom you have given their dowries, and those whom your right hand possesses out of those whom Allah has given to you as prisoners of war, *and the daughters of your paternal uncles and the daughters of your paternal aunts, and the daughters of your maternal uncles and the daughters of your maternal aunts who fled with you; and a believing woman if she gave herself to the Prophet, if the Prophet desired to marry her—<u>specially for you, not for the (rest of) believers;</u> We know what We have ordained for them concerning their wives and those whom their right hands possess in order that no blame may attach to you; and Allah is Forgiving, Merciful. (33:50)*

With these words, Muhammad used God to give himself permission to use all methods at his disposal to satisfy his insatiable sexual appetite. The *Quran* also says:

مَّا كَانَ عَلَى النَّبِيِّ مِنْ حَرَجٍ فِيمَا فَرَضَ اللَّهُ لَهُ سُنَّةَ اللَّهِ فِي الَّذِينَ خَلَوْا مِن قَبْلُ وَكَانَ أَمْرُ اللَّهِ قَدَرًا مَّقْدُورًا

There is no harm in the Prophet doing that which Allah has ordained for him; such has been the course of Allah with respect to those who have gone before; and the command of Allah is a decree that is made absolute. (33:38)

Muhammad thus used the *Quran* as a method of rationalization to justify and gratify his own inner needs and desires. This type of situation created a great deal of headaches for Muhammad's devout followers, who were now forced to use additional rationalizations to justify his behaviors. Through the *Quran,* Muhammad could tell others what he would not say himself—for with God saying it, there would be no shame upon him.

The following verse is another good example of this method. Muhammad used to let his followers come to his home to eat supper and listen to him preach. He and his followers would then spend the evening talking. After a while, this became too much for Muhammad,

PERSONALITY CHANGES: HYPER-RELIGIOSITY AND SEXUAL BEHAVIORS

so he had to find a polite way out. He used the following verse to deliver to himself:

يا أَيُّها الَّذِينَ آمَنُوا لَا تَدْخُلُوا بُيُوتَ النَّبِيِّ إِلَّا أَن يُؤْذَنَ لَكُمْ إِلَى طَعَامٍ غَيْرَ نَاظِرِينَ إِنَاهُ وَلَٰكِنْ إِذَا دُعِيتُمْ فَادْخُلُوا فَإِذَا طَعِمْتُمْ فَانتَشِرُوا وَلَا مُسْتَأْنِسِينَ لِحَدِيثٍ إِنَّ ذَٰلِكُمْ كَانَ يُؤْذِي النَّبِيَّ فَيَسْتَحْيِي مِنكُمْ وَاللَّهُ لَا يَسْتَحْيِي مِنَ الْحَقِّ وَإِذَا سَأَلْتُمُوهُنَّ مَتَاعًا فَاسْأَلُوهُنَّ مِن وَرَاءِ حِجَابٍ ذَٰلِكُمْ أَطْهَرُ

O you who believe! Do not enter the houses of the Prophet unless permission is given to you for a meal, not waiting for its cooking being finished—but when you are invited, enter, and when you have taken the food, then disperse—not seeking to listen to talk; surely this gives the Prophet trouble, but he forbears from you, and Allah does not forbear from the truth. And when you ask of them any goods, ask of them from behind a curtain; this is purer for your hearts and (for) their hearts; and it does not behoove you that you should give trouble to the Messenger of Allah, nor that you should marry his wives after him ever; surely this is grievous in the sight of Allah. (33:53)

Muhammad's appetite for beautiful women was evident again after the war of Banu Mostalagh, one of his last battles. Many prisoners had been taken, some of whom offered to buy their freedom. In cases in which the price was set too high, the prisoners were brought before Muhammad to make their case. One such prisoner was a beautiful woman.

Aysha is quoted as saying that she knew the woman was trouble as soon as she laid eyes on her, simply because she was attractive and Muhammad would want her for himself. She was right. Muhammad offered to pay the bounty to make the woman free if she would agree to become his wife. Her captor refused to take the money but granted her freedom anyway, thereby forging a bond with Muhammad. Seeing that the woman's imprisoned family members were now related by marriage to the clan of Muhammad, the captors freed all of the prisoners.

SWORD AND SEIZURE

Defenders of Muhammad claim that this had been his intention all along. However, given what we know of Muhammad's relationships, it is more likely that he was motivated solely by desire for the woman. After all, if he wanted to set all the prisoners free, he could have done so without marrying the young woman. In the final analysis, Muhammad was the Prophet and his word was the law, and he did not fear making unpopular decisions.

THE STORY OF ZEINAB

Another strange example of Muhammad's seemingly boundless sexual appetites is the story of Zeinab, the woman who married Muhammad's adopted son, Zayd. Zayd was a former slave whom Muhammad's wife Khadijeh gave to him when Zayd was very young. Muhammad was so fond of him that he freed the child and adopted him as his own son. Zayd and Ali, Muhammad's cousin, were later to become the Prophet's two closest companions.

When Zayd became a young man, Muhammad was determined to find a wife for him. He decided that Zayd would marry his cousin Zeinab, who was an attractive young woman. For her part, Zeinab did not like the idea of a union with Zayd; after all, he was merely an adopted and freed slave. Further, Zayd did not have a large family, which was a quality considered important in spousal selection. In the end, it was probably the prominence and influence of Muhammad that convinced Zeinab to consent to the marriage.

But things went awry quickly for the young couple. One month into the marriage, Muhammad went to visit his adopted son. Zayd was not home; instead, Zeinab answered the door, dressed rather skimpily. Muhammad suddenly saw his beautiful young cousin in a whole new light. He is said to have exclaimed to her, "You are attractive and you also steal one's heart!"

The short chance encounter was the beginning of the end for the marriage. When Zayd later heard the story from Zeinab, he quickly

Personality Changes: Hyper-Religiosity and Sexual Behaviors

decided to hand over the subject of his adopted father's desire. He went to Muhammad and pledged to divorce Zeinab and give her to him to marry. But Muhammad refused the offer, telling Zayd to "go home, fear Allah, and take care of your wife." A few days later, Zayd made the offer again, and again received the same response from Muhammad.

The problem for Muhammad was not just that it was unseemly for the Prophet to take somebody else's wife out of passion. The laws of the time strictly prohibited a father to marry his son's wife after divorce or death. This was true even when that son was adopted—all of the rules of a natural son or daughter applied. In this situation, the law recognized Zayd, the adopted son, as no different from natural born sons. Therefore, Zeinab was totally prohibited to Muhammad.

But when Zayd brought the offer to Muhammad for a third time, things suddenly changed. Several *ayahs* came upon the Prophet, and he began to receive a message from God. In these verses, God chastised Muhammad for being shy and reluctant to report His word, telling Muhammad that god has changed the law prohibiting marriage to a son's wife.

Zayd was commanded to divorce Zeinab immediately, and she was pledged to marry Muhammad after the customary 100-day grace period had passed. On the one hundredth day after the divorce, Muhammad, in an uncharacteristic hurry, is said to have rushed into Zeinab's home, married her immediately and had sex with her that night. Zeinab quickly became one of Muhammad's four favorite wives.

Today, many Muslim clerics justify Muhammad's actions by reasoning that God used the Prophet in order to abolish the old pagan rules against marrying the wife of one's son. However, if this were true, could not God have simply given that order and save Muhammad from so much controversy? It seems more likely that Muhammad used the vehicle of the *Quran* to make the rules that suited his needs.

وَإِذْ تَقُولُ لِلَّذِي أَنْعَمَ اللَّهُ عَلَيْهِ وَأَنْعَمْتَ عَلَيْهِ أَمْسِكْ عَلَيْكَ زَوْجَكَ وَاتَّقِ اللَّهَ وَتُخْفِي فِي نَفْسِكَ مَا اللَّهُ مُبْدِيهِ وَتَخْشَى النَّاسَ وَاللَّهُ أَحَقُّ أَنْ تَخْشَاهُ فَلَمَّا قَضَى زَيْدٌ مِنْهَا وَطَراً زَوَّجْنَاكَهَا لِكَيْ لَا يَكُونَ عَلَى الْمُؤْمِنِينَ حَرَجٌ فِي أَزْوَاجِ أَدْعِيَائِهِمْ إِذَا قَضَوْا مِنْهُنَّ وَطَراً وَكَانَ أَمْرُ اللَّهِ مَفْعُولًا

And when you said to him to whom Allah had shown favor and to whom you had shown a favor: Keep your wife to yourself and be careful of (your duty to) Allah; and you concealed in your soul what Allah would bring to light, and you feared men, and Allah had a greater right that you should fear him. But when Zayd had accomplished his want of her, we gave her to you as a wife, so that there should be no difficulty for the believers in respect of the wives of their adopted sons, when they have accomplished their want of them; and Allah's command shall be performed. (The *Quran*, 33:37)

This is one of the great examples of the changes that occurred in Muhammad's behavior after he developed the seizures. After all, it is common knowledge that most men become less sexually active after the age of 50, not more so. Yet in his late fifties, Muhammad behaved sexually more like an adolescent. The story of Zeinab also clearly shows how Muhammad used the *Quran* to gratify his inner needs. Because we know that he would have never done such a thing consciously, this is a good indication that most of these processes were at an unconscious level and that he did not have much insight into his seizure-induced behaviors.

When a cousin of Aysha, Muhammad's most favorite wife, came to visit her while Muhammad was not home, the Prophet became angry at the man. He warned him against such visits, but the man declared his innocence, insisting that the woman was only a cousin and the visit had been purely platonic. When Muhammad again chastised him, the man made an offhand comment to the effect of, "Well, anyway, you're old and when you die I'll marry her." Not surprisingly, there was soon another law, recorded in verse 53 of the *sura* "Ahzab," in which it was written that no one could marry Muhammad's wives after his death, as this would upset him in the afterlife.

ولا أن تنكِحُوا أَزْواجَهُ مِن بعْدِه أبدا إنَّ ذلكُمْ كان عند اللّه عظيما

Do not marry his wives after him ever. Surely this is grievous in the sight of Allah. (33:53)

Conclusions Regarding Muhammad's Behaviors

The *Quran* is meant to be a religious book. Critics agree that while the *Quran* should reflect some connections to Muhammad's life as it fit into the context of his mission and the turbulent times, it should not read so much like a soap opera. What does this tell us about Muhammad's psyche? The hypersexuality that overtook him as a result of complex partial seizures also took over a large portion of his life. Sex became such a major part of his thinking that it became a part of the *Quran*.

To use Freudian terminology, Muhammad's hypersexuality, which resulted from his seizure disorder, intensified his inner conflicts. The strength of his instincts became so powerful that he was not capable of controlling his desires and had to resort to childish rationalizations to justify them. It is in this light that we can understand why a holy man would devise a rule that stated no one but him could have more than four wives. But Muhammad did not stop with rules for the living—his possessiveness of his wives prompted him to establish laws that extended beyond the grave.

Muhammad's sexuality clearly had a major impact on his personal life and on his mission. Although there are many other examples and illustrations of his sexual pursuits, the above examples adequately document the changes in this aspect of his life pursuant to the beginning of his seizures.

CHAPTER 6

PERSONALITY CHANGES: AGGRESSION

إنما جزاء الذين يحاربون الله ورسوله ويسعون في الأرض فسادًا أن يقتلوا أو يصلبوا أو تقطع أيديهم وأرجلهم من خلاف أو ينفوا من الأرض ذلك لهم خزي في الدنيا ولهم في الآخرة عذاب عظيم

The punishment of those who wage war against Allah and His Messenger, and strive with might and main for mischief through the land is: execution, or crucifixion, or the cutting off of hands and feet from opposite sides, or exile from the land: that is their disgrace in this world, and a heavy punishment is theirs in the Hereafter;

—Quran, 5:33

Throughout Muhammad's early years, he is not known as being an aggressive person. During his childhood, he was an orphan who was known for being quiet and introspective. When he was about 15 years old, Muhammad participated in the wars of Fajar, which lasted approximately five years. Muhammad told many people that his job during the war was to help his uncles and his clan by collecting arrows for the archers, although it has been reported that he might have held the position of an archer toward the end of the war. The wars of Fajar were most likely a beneficial event in Muhammad's life, as he was able to learn the tactics of war. However, he did not gain the reputation of being violent or warrior-like at the time.

MUHAMMAD'S LIFE OF NON-AGGRESSION

Muhammad spent most of his young life as a merchant, and there are no reports that he was aggressive or got into trouble during his twenties or thirties. Muhammad spent the years between the ages of 40 and 50 peacefully preaching Islam and recruiting and teaching his followers. Muhammad's main desire in life during this time was to be introspective and introverted, and he passively tolerated any ridicule or harassment. There are many reports that he was a quiet person who would not talk excessively and that he liked ritualistic prayers the best.

The fact that Muhammad was not an aggressive person made him a target of abuse during the first years of Islam. Muhammad had a cousin by the name of Hamza who was a hunter and a warrior. Hamza converted to Islam early in Muhammad's ministry, and his conversion provided the strong protection that Muhammad could not provide for himself. From the period of time between Muhammad introducing himself as a prophet to his migration to Medina, there was still no overt sign of aggressive behavior.

Although Muhammad's uncles and his clan provided him and his well-to-do followers with some protection, those of his followers who did not have status had no protection of any kind (Ibn Ishaq, P143). Many of these followers were tortured and killed, but Muhammad still did not show any significant aggressive retaliatory behavior. Even the early parts of the *Quran* contain many verses promoting patience and tolerance (*sura* 103). *Valathr* is one of those sections of the *Quran*:

والْعَصْرُ

I swear by the time,

إنّ الْإنسان لفي خُسْر

Most surely man is in loss,

إلّا الّذين آمنوا وعملوا الصّالحات وتواصوْا بالْحقّ وتواصوْا بالصّبْر

Except those who believe and do good, and enjoin on each other truth, and enjoin on each other patience. (103:1–3)

Another section of the *Quran* written during Muhammad's early years in Mecca that promotes kindness is *sura* 90, "Al-Balad" (the Arabic in these parts of the *Quran* is extremely beautiful):

لَا أُقْسِمُ بِهَذَا الْبَلَدِ

Nay! I swear by this city.

وَأَنتَ حِلٌّ بِهَذَا الْبَلَدِ

And you shall be made free from obligation in this city—

وَوَالِدٍ وَمَا وَلَدَ

And the begetter and whom he begot.

لَقَدْ خَلَقْنَا الْإِنسَانَ فِي كَبَدٍ

Certainly we have created man to be in distress.

أَيَحْسَبُ أَن لَّن يَقْدِرَ عَلَيْهِ أَحَدٌ

Does he think that no one has power over him?

يَقُولُ أَهْلَكْتُ مَالًا لُّبَدًا

He shall say: "I have wasted much wealth."

أَيَحْسَبُ أَن لَّمْ يَرَهُ أَحَدٌ

Does he think that no one sees him?

أَلَمْ نَجْعَل لَّهُ عَيْنَيْنِ

Have we not given him two eyes,

وَلِسَانًا وَشَفَتَيْنِ

And a tongue and two lips,

و هديْناهُ النَّجْديْن

And pointed out to him the two conspicuous ways?

فلا اقْتحم الْعقبة

But he would not attempt the uphill road,

وما أدْراك ما الْعقبة

And what will make you comprehend what the uphill road is?

فكُّ رقبة

[It is] the setting free of a slave,

أوْ إطْعامٌ في يوْمٍ ذي مسْغبة

Or the giving of food in a day of hunger

يتيما ذا مقْربة

To an orphan, having relationship,

أوْ مسْكينا ذا متْربة

Or to the poor man lying in the dust.

ثمَّ كان من الَّذين آمنوا وتواصوْا بالصَّبْر وتواصوْا بالْمرْحمة

Then he is of those who believe and charge one another to show patience, and charge one another to show compassion.

أوْلئك أصْحابُ الْميْمنة

These are the people of the right hand.

والَّذين كفرُوا بآياتنا هُمْ أصْحابُ المشْأمة

And [as for] those who disbelieve in our communications, they are the people of the left hand.

عَلَيْهِمْ نَارٌ مُّؤْصَدَةٌ

On them is fire closed over.

THE MIGRATION TO MEDINA

Things did not really begin to change for Muhammad until 10 years after his claim to prophethood. That year, a contingent from the city of Yathreb (a city in competition with Mecca) arrived in Mecca to take part in the annual washing of the idols and general maintenance of the Kaaba. The annual event was a golden opportunity for Muhammad to preach in relative safety. Killing was strictly forbidden in the vicinity of the Kaaba, and never more so than during these holy festivals. Muhammad could preach and recruit uninhibited, and he took full advantage of the situation. It happened that in his tenth year of preaching, the visitors from Yathreb were receptive to his message.

The people of Yathreb had many problems of their own at home. Although the city of Yathreb, the second largest city in Arabia, was an oasis with a milder climate and more fertile farmland than Mecca, it was also the site of much tribal feud. Most of the Yathreb tribes were either pagan or Jewish. The pagan tribes tended to be poor and were often engaged in fierce (and frequently deadly) internal squabbling. The Jewish tribes tended to be wealthier and frequently employed Arabs to work their farmland. For this reason, the people of Yathreb were anxious for conflicts to be resolved. They had heard of Muhammad's intellect and his superior negotiating skills.

When the contingent visiting Mecca heard the Prophet's ideas and his preaching, they were impressed enough to bring a larger group the following year. Seventy men and women traveled to Mecca for the pilgrimage and to meet with the Prophet. After some discussions, the contingent from Yathreb invited Muhammad to immigrate to their city and live under the protection of its people. A treaty was drafted and signed, and Muhammad and his followers moved to Yathreb.

All of this happened none too soon, for the controversial prophet had long since worn out his welcome in Mecca. The pagans in the city had resolved at last to kill him and pay for the revenge. It was only through the efforts of his cousin Ali that Muhammad was able to escape from the city unharmed. At the time of migration, or *Hejrah*, Muhammad was 53 years old, 13 years after his first encounter with the angel Gabriel in the cave of Hira.

Muhammad's departure from Mecca created uproar. An angry mob took off after him and his traveling companion, Abu Baker (later his successor). The two barely completed the 300-mile journey to Yathreb in one piece. Once in Yathreb, however, they were greeted warmly. Shortly after Muhammad's arrival, the city's official name was changed to Madinah Al Nabi, which literally means the "the city of prophet." Muhammad was to live out the rest of his life in Medina. Upon his death there 10 years later, the year of his migration became the first year of the Islamic calendar, marking the beginning of Islam's transformation from a local faith to an international religion.

Muhammad's move to Medina also marked an important transformation in the Prophet's life. Muhammad was no longer a street-corner preacher and self-proclaimed prophet but a statesman and revered holy man. Not surprisingly, with the combination of his new responsibilities and the progression of his disease, his behavior began to change at this time.

One of the greatest changes in Muhammad's life was that he now had help in spreading his message, as greater numbers of people had begun to accept and embrace his teachings. Muhammad's enemies gradually began to recognize him as a force to be reckoned with, and his confidence soon grew. Muhammad believed that he was God's true messenger and, as such, declared that everyone who was against him was also against God. And while Muhammad recognized the importance of the prophets who had come before him, he placed himself above all others, claiming that God had given him alone the authority to make decisions in God's name.

JIHAD: THE DOCTRINE OF VIOLENCE

One of the changes in the Prophet's behavior was the introduction of war and violence into his doctrine. He began to war against his enemies and their rich caravans and to send his followers on dangerous missions of piracy and assassination. In fact, one of the main reasons why Muhammad was able to get rid of most of his enemies in such a short time was the fact that he was very good at war. He had the characteristics of a good general. He made excellent use of espionage and assassinated those who stood in his way.

As with all patients who suffer with complex partial seizures, Muhammad had a profound sense of his purpose in life. Muhammad's mission, as he saw it, was to spread the message that Allah was the one and only God and that he, Muhammad, was his chosen messenger. He could have attempted to accomplish this mission by continuing to preach peace, tolerance and patience. But given the new power that he experienced in Medina, Muhammad instead chose to adopt a much more forceful approach. Had he stayed on the path he had been on in Mecca, he would have likely been remembered as just another prophet among many. The world might never have known him as Muhammad, the founder of Islam and father of the one of the largest religions on Earth.

But even as Muhammad's star was rising in Medina, his health began to deteriorate. His seizures became more frequent and he began to receive "visits" from the angel Gabriel almost daily. (There is better documentation of the occurrence of seizures when Muhammad was in Medina because there were many more people around Muhammad to witness them.) The pressures of having to deliver on so many promises weighed heavily on Muhammad. Even his new followers were becoming restless. It is said that when pagan armies surrounded Medina during the famous Battle of Trench, one of Muhammad's followers complained, "Muhammad promises the treasure of Persia and Rome, but here we cannot go to the bathroom in peace!" (Al Waqedy, 1986, Persian translation, 3:345).

Muhammad clearly needed an infusion of resources in order to fulfill his vision for his people. In other words, he had to wage war and inevitably he and his followers would have to kill. But for death to be accepted among his followers, Muhammad knew that he would have to change the rules of engagement.

It was at this crucial point that the verses of the *Quran* relating to *jihad* (literally meaning "struggle" in Arabic—most similar to the term "crusade" in the Christian world) were added to the sacred text. According to Muhammad, anyone killed in a war sanctioned by the Prophet would go directly to heaven; all others would be subject to Judgment Day. Since according to Muhammad the only residents of heaven prior to Judgment Day were Allah, his angels and the prophets, saints and martyrs, a one-way ticket to heaven was enormously appealing for Muslims.

The early years of Islam in Medina had been difficult for Muhammad and his followers, most of whom had to resort to low-level manual labor just to survive. Housing was minimal and food was scarce. Even Muhammad himself sometimes went to bed on an empty stomach. However, once his campaigns against caravans traveling between Mecca and Syria began, Muhammad and his followers gradually began to reap the rewards.

Once this new, more aggressive doctrine had been laid out, Muhammad began to condone behaviors that he had never sanctioned in Mecca. The spoils of larger and larger battles included weapons, camels, horses, jewels, money, and, most importantly, prisoners of war. These prisoners were often sold back to their families or into slavery, and thus represented an important source of income. Many of Muhammad's followers became so enamored with the concept of *jihad* and the possibility of eternal salvation that they would implore him to pray for their

Personality Changes: Aggression

death in battle. Muhammad's portrait of heaven, painted so eloquently after his own ascension experience, was so enticing and appealing that his followers were literally "dying" to go. After all, who wouldn't trade the hot, arid deserts of Arabia for the promise of peace and freedom in the lush gardens of God? In contrast to the Christian heaven, wherein the devout continue to praise and worship God, Muslims are promised a good time in the afterlife. Even wine, forbidden to Muhammad's followers on earth, was said to flow freely in the rivers of heaven.

Muhammad's first major battle with his pagan enemy was a rousing success. His bedraggled band of 300 men defeated 1,000 well-equipped soldiers. The victory brought him the fame and notoriety given to all great soldiers and also helped him to solidify his cause, recruit new followers, and set his sights on greater conquests.

An eloquent speaker with an impressive vocabulary, Muhammad told the tale of each victory over and over, embellishing where necessary for the greatest effect. Muhammad told his rapt audiences that Allah and 1,000 angels were behind them, carrying them to victory over seemingly more powerful enemies. Fighting on Muhammad's side was a win-win situation—if a soldier was victorious in battle, the spoils were his reward; but if a soldier died in battle, heaven awaited. These promises propelled Muhammad's forces to conquer most of the world that was then known to Arabs. In fact, Muhammad had a winning streak almost unparalleled in history; he was victorious in all but one battle.

It was not only the motivation of *jihad* and martyrdom that granted Muhammad so many victories. He was also a clever strategist, skilled at espionage, and adept at pitting his enemies against each other. By the end of his life, Muhammad's army was so large and strong that they were able to go up against the Roman Empire with a force of 10,000 men.

The booty that Muhammad's forces gained from these wars was an enormous source of income and weaponry for future battles. Unfortunately, although Muhammad proposed proper and fair treatment of captives, he did not outlaw the habit of taking slaves—a fact that caused future generations to become strong proponents of slave trading.

Even today, there are slaves and slave traders in some Islamic countries in North Africa (The African Commission on Human and Peoples' Rights 2004).

To Muhammad, freeing slaves was simply good manners, but not a mandatory compulsion. There are numerous reports that he made enormous amounts of money by taking captives. He also received one-fifth of the profits that his followers made from selling captives. From the booty taken during a war, Muhammad went so far in this behavior as to permit his followers to take female captives to their homes for sex, regardless of whether the women were married—the marriage of a woman who was married to an infidel and was captured in battle was considered null and void (Dashti [Persian], 205).

WARS AGAINST THE JEWS AND PAGANS

Muhammad's violent behaviors in Medina are in total contrast to his preaching of kindness and tolerance during the Mecca years. His transformation from a peaceful merchant into a hardened general is too profound to be a byproduct of becoming a statesman; the driving factors are undoubtedly influenced by the progression of the disease.

There were three Jewish tribes in Medina who were at odds with the Arab tribes. The Jews were rich and educated, while the Arabs were poor (and mostly worked for the Jews). Muhammad bitterly disliked the Jews of Arabia. He believed that Jews were hypocrites. He was reported as saying that "the Jewish people are waiting for the Messiah to come, and now that the Messiah has arrived, they should be the first to accept him." But the Jewish tribes did not accept Muhammad as a prophet of God, which bothered him immensely.

In a battle in A.D. 625, Muhammad defeated the Jewish tribe of Qaynuqa, took their wealth, and kicked them out of Medina, permitting them only to take their portable wealth. Through this action, Muhammad was able to get a great deal of land, palm trees, and housing for himself and his followers. The members of the Jewish tribe that

PERSONALITY CHANGES: AGGRESSION

Muhammad defeated later went to a Jewish area of Arabia, adopted the name Khaibar, and continued to conspire against him.

During the first few years that Muhammad lived in Medina, he had several serious battles with the pagans. He was able to survive these wars, win a few battles, and generally make a name for himself throughout Arabia. In A.D. 627, he faced the greatest of these battles, the Battle of the Trench. The pagan tribes, which had now been defeated several times, were able to unite and raise an army of 10,000 men to attack Muhammad in Medina.

Before the pagan army arrived at the gates of Medina, Muhammad managed to make a non-aggression treaty with the last Jewish tribe of Medina, the Banu Qurayza. Muhammad was worried that the Banu Qurayza would help the pagans from inside the city, and he knew that there was no way he could fight on two fronts. For their part, the Banu Qurayza did not want to have a fate similar to the Qaynuqa, and so they signed a peace treaty with Muhammad to avoid annihilation.

The pagans surrounded Medina for several weeks but could not break through the trench around the city. The pagans therefore negotiated with the reluctant Banu Qurayza and persuaded them to attack Muhammad's army from both inside and outside the city. However, Muhammad was able to create conflict between the two forces, and the alliance between the pagans and the Banu Qurayza soon failed. Eventually, the pagans got tired of waiting in the desert and retreated to their cities, leaving the Jews alone in Medina with an angry Muhammad and his followers.

On the same day that the pagans left, Muhammad began a war against the Banu Qurayza. Ibn Ishaq reported this event as follows:

> According to what Al-Zuhri told me, at the time of the noon prayers Gabriel came to the apostle wearing an embroidered turban and riding on a mule with a saddle covered with a piece of brocade. He asked the apostle if he had abandoned fighting, and when he said that he had, he said that the angels had not yet laid aside their arms and that he had just come from pursuing

the enemy. "God commands you, Muhammad, to go to [Banu] Qurayza. I am about to go to them to shake their stronghold." (Ibn Ishaq, P 461)

Muhammad called on his followers to go to war against the Banu Qurayza. They besieged the Jewish area for three weeks and finally set fire to their palm trees. At that point, the Jewish leaders gave up and surrendered. They asked Muhammad to treat them the same way he had treated the Qaynuqa, hoping that he would allow them leave in peace. However, Muhammad did not agree, and after some further negotiation, the Jewish leaders allowed a third-party of Muhammad's choosing to decide their fate. The third-party that Muhammad chose was Sad b. Muadh, one of the leaders of the Arab tribes of Medina, who naturally sided with Muhammad and ordered that the Jewish men be decapitated, and the women and children to be taken into captivity. The following report of this event, as told by Ibn Ishaq, is the version most agreed upon by historians:

> Then the apostle went out to the market of Medina . . . and dug trenches in it. Then he sent for them and struck off their heads in those trenches as they were brought out to him in batches. Among them was the enemy of Allah Huyayy b. Akhtab and Ka'b b. Asad their chief. There were 600 or 700 in all, though some put the figure as high as 800 or 900. As they were being taken out in batches to the apostle they asked Ka'b what he thought would be done with them. He replied, "Will you never understand? Don't you see that the summoner never stops and those who are taken away do not return? By Allah it is death!" This went on until the apostle made an end of them. (Ibn Ishaq, P 465)

The decapitations took about one-and-one-half days to complete. The executioners included Ali, Muhammad's cousin, and Zayd,

Personality Changes: Aggression

Muhammad's stepson. The Jews' wealth was confiscated and their women and children were sold into slavery, except for one woman:

> Muhammad b. Ja'far b. al-Zubayr told me from Urwa b. al-Zubayr that Ayesha said: "Only one of their women was killed. She was actually with me and was talking with me and laughing immoderately as the apostle was killing her men in the market when suddenly an unseen voice called her name. 'Good heavens,' I cried, 'what is the matter?' 'I am to be killed,' she replied. 'What for?' I asked. 'Because of something I did,' she answered." She was taken away and beheaded. Ayesha used to say, "I when all the time she knew that she would be killed." She was the woman who threw a millstone down from the Qurayza fort and killed a believer. (Ibn Ishaq, P465)

Some of Muhammad's biographers try to rationalize his behavior by saying that it was caused by his fear for his faith and his followers. They suggest that Muhammad feared that if he did not fight hard, his enemies would kill him and his followers in one swift savage killing—a genuine concern during those times. However, this is only a justification, because the Prophet and his followers' total annihilation was always a possibility during the years he lived in Mecca as well as the first few years he lived in Medina. His brutal behavior only sprang up in Medina when he had the internal change and the external following to be able to act out on his aggressive impulses. Somehow every defeat or tie was followed with a lucrative attack on the Jewish tribes! His life became consumed with conquering his enemies, making his followers happy, gaining glory in the Arabic lands, and punishing those who would not listen.

Assassinations

Some of Muhammad's aggressive behaviors after his migration to Medina are simply too brutal and odd to match his character of just a few years before. Muhammad utilized political assassination to deal with his staunchest enemies. He sent his devout followers after people who ridiculed him or conspired against him, especially those who questioned his prophethood.

Sallam Ibn Abu'l-Huqayq was a Jewish leader living in the fortresses of Khaibar, the last stronghold of the Jews in Arabia. When the fighting at the trench and the affair of the Banu Qurayza were over, the matter of Sallam Ibn Abu'l-Huqayq, known as the Abu Rafi, came up in connection with those who had instigated and brought the tribes together against Muhammad.

> Now Aus had killed Ka'b b. al-Ashraf before Uhud because of his enmity towards Muhammad and because he instigated men against him, so Khazraj asked and obtained the apostle's permission to kill Sallam who was in Khaibar. Muhammad b. Muslim b. Shihab al-Zuhri from Abdullah b. Ka'b b. Malik told me: "One of the things which God did for His apostle was that these two tribes of the Ansar [original tribes of Medina], Aus, and Khazraj competed the one with the other like two stallions: If Aus did anything to the apostle's advantage, Khazraj would say, 'They shall not have this superiority over us in the apostle's eyes and in Islam' and they would not rest until they could do something similar. If Khazraj did anything, Aus would say the same.
>
> When Aus had killed Ka'b for his enmity towards the apostle, Khazraj used these words and asked themselves what man was as hostile to the apostle as Ka'b? And then they remembered Sallam who was in Khaibar and asked and obtained the apostle's permission to kill him.
>
> Five men of B. Salima of Khazraj went to him: Abdullah b. 'Atik; Mas'ud b. Sinan; 'Abdullah b. Unays; Abu Qatada al-Hartith b. Rib'i; and Khuza'i b. Aswad, an ally from Aslam. As they left, the apostle appointed 'Abdullah b. 'Atik as their leader, and

Personality Changes: Aggression

he forbade them to kill women or children. When they got to Khaibar they went to Sallam's house by night, having locked every door in the settlement on the inhabitants. Now he was in an upper chamber of his to which a ladder led up. They mounted this until they came to the door and asked to be allowed to come in. His wife came out and asked who they were and they told her that they were Arabs in search of supplies. She told them that their man was here and that they could come in. When we entered, we bolted the door of the room on her and ourselves fearing lest something should come between us and him. His wife shrieked and warned him of us, so we ran at him with our swords, as he was on his bed. The only thing that guided us in the darkness of the night was his whiteness like an Egyptian blanket. When his wife shrieked one of our number he would lift his sword against her; then he would remember the apostle's ban on killing women and withdraw his hand; but for that we would have made an end of her that night. When we had smitten him with our swords, 'Abdullah b. Unays bore down with his sword into his belly until it went right through him, as he was saying, 'Qatni, qatni,' i.e., 'it's enough, enough.'

We went out. Now 'Abdullah b. 'Atik had poor sight and fell from the ladder and sprained his arm severely, so we carried him until we brought him to one of their water channels and went into it. The people lit lamps and went in search of us in all directions until, despairing of finding us, they returned to their master and gathered round him as he was dying. We asked each other how we could know that the enemy of God was dead, and one of us volunteered to go and see; so off he went and mingled with the people. He said, 'I found his wife and some Jews gathered round him. She had a lamp in her hand and was peering into his face and saying to them, 'By God, I certainly heard the voice of 'Abdullah b. 'Atik. Then I decided I must be wrong and thought, *How can Ibn 'Atik be in this country?'*

Then she turned towards him, looking into his face, and said, 'By the God of the Jews he is dead!' Never have I heard sweeter words than those.

Then he came to us and told us the news, and we picked up our companion and took him to the apostle and told him that we had killed God's enemy. We disputed before him as to who had killed him, each of us laying claim to the deed. The apostle demanded to see our swords and when he looked at them he said, 'It is the sword of 'Abdullah b. Unays that killed him; I can see traces of food on it.'" (Ibn Ishaq, 482–483)

Looking into Muhammad's life, we find about half dozen of these assassinations. Most of the assassins that he chose were people of poor character before converting to Islam and devout followers afterwards.

There is a list of people that Muhammad ordered to be killed in Mecca when he conquered the city. As mentioned earlier, Mecca was considered a sacred area; no one was allowed to kill anybody or anything around the city. This was the law before Muhammad arrived, and he kept the rule (it still stands today). However, a few of his enemies made him so angry that he broke the rule and ordered them to be killed.

Muhammad even broke one of his own rules regarding the killing of women by ordering the assassination of two women singers who had written bad songs about him. The story goes this way:

'Abdullah b. Chantal of B. Tam b. Ghazi had become a Muslim and the Apostle sent him to collect the poor tax in company with one of the Amstar. He had with him a freed slave who served him. (He was a Muslim.) When they halted, he ordered the latter to kill a goat for him and prepare some food and went to sleep. When he woke up, the man had done nothing, so he attacked and killed him and apostatized. He had two singing-girls, Fortuna and her friend, who used to sing songs about the

Apostle, so he ordered that they should be killed with him. (Ibn Ishaq, P 551)

TORTURE

Muhammad is also known for ordering beatings and torture. It should be noted that this "torture" does not refer to physical punishments that Islam permits as a part of a person's sentence for Islamic wrongdoings, such as flogging for drinking alcohol or cutting off a hand in the case of burglary. Rather, the torture that Muhammad ordered was for the purpose of obtaining information from people who did not want to talk.

When Muhammad was 60 years old and in the final years of his life, he initiated a war against the last Jewish tribes of Arabia. At that time, following a series of wars, most of the Jews in western Arabia had been driven to a colony of fortresses in Khaibar. In the past, Muhammad had gone to war against these tribes for a multitude of reasons. In this instance, the reason was because of a truce that Muhammad had signed with the pagans. The terms of this treaty favored the pagans, and Muhammad's most devoted followers began openly criticizing him for signing such a demeaning treaty. So Muhammad, in a few weeks, took his army to Khaibar to fight the Jews, knowing that a victory in this battlefield would satisfy his followers' need for victory, money, and prestige. His attack was so sudden that he took the Jews by total surprise and was able to open the castles one by one. In the last castle, he found the leader of the tribes.

Muhammad knew that there was gold, diamonds and rubies hidden somewhere in the castle, as the profession of some of these tribes was goldsmithing. However, the leader of the Jews, Kinana, would not reveal the location of the treasure, so Muhammad ordered him to be tortured until he talked. Muhammad then ordered Kinana to be decapitated and confiscated his wealth, took his wife (who was only 17 years old at the time) for himself as a wife, and sold the rest of his family into slavery.

It is said that Allah Almighty guided the Prophet (PBUH) to where the treasure was . . . When the treasure had been dug up, the Prophet (PBUH) ordered Zubayr to torture Kinana Ibnu Abu AlHuqaiq to extract everything from him. Zubayr obeyed and tortured him to the point of plunging a bone in his chest. The Prophet (PBUH) then ordered that he be handed to Muhammad Ibnu Maslama to kill him and his brother. Muhammad Ibnu Maslama killed him and ordered that his brother be tortured. After that, he handed him to the relatives of Bistro Ibnu Albarraa, and they killed him. Some say he was decapitated. The Prophet (PBUH) declared the confiscation of their wealth lawful and imprisoned their progeny. (Al Waghedy, Persian translation, 1986, 2:512)

In a related incident during approximately same time period, Muhammad and his son-in-law Ali were involved in an unpleasant event. Apparently, Muhammad's young, beautiful, and mouthy wife Aysha was accused of infidelity, and they were trying to get to the truth of the matter. When Muhammad asked Ali's opinion on the situation, he said:

"Women are plentiful, and you can easily change one for another. Ask the slave girl, for she will tell you the truth." So the Apostle called Burayra to ask her, and Ali got up and gave her a violent beating, saying, "Tell the Apostle the truth," to which she replied, "I know only good of her." (Ibn Ishaq, P496)

Other incidents in which Muhammad ordered or authorized torture in order to obtain military information or for other purposes are also well documented.

CHAPTER 7

THE NIGHT JOURNEY: MEERAJ

Then the apostle was carried by night from the mosque at Mecca to the Masjid al-Aqsa, which is the temple of Aelia, when Islam had spread in Mecca between the Ghouraish and all the tribes.
—Ibn Ishaq, P181

There is perhaps no better window into the unconscious mind of Muhammad than the story of his ascension into heaven. The story, while extraordinary, has caused much controversy throughout history and is probably the least understood episode in the Prophet's life.

THE JOURNEY TO HEAVEN

Not long after Muhammad claimed to be the prophet of Allah, he had a strange and powerful dream. In his dream, the angel Gabriel came to him and escorted him on an incredible journey into the heavens. Here is the story from Muhammad, as reported by Ibn Ishaq:

> The apostle said: "While I was sleeping in the Hijr, Gabriel came and stirred me with his foot. I sat up but saw nothing and lay

down again. He came down again. He came to me the third time and stirred me with his foot.

I sat up and he took hold of my arm and I stood beside him; and he brought me out to the door of the mosque and there was a white animal, half mule, half donkey, with wings on its sides with which it propelled its feet, putting each forefoot at the limit of its sight and he mounted me on it. Then he went out with me, keeping close to me.

The Apostle said: "When I came up to mount him, he shied. Gabriel placed his hand on its mane and said, 'Are you not ashamed, O Buraq, to behave in this way? By God, none more honorable before God than Muhammad has ever ridden you before.' The animal was so ashamed that he broke out into a sweat and stood still so that I could mount him." The apostle and Gabriel went their way until they arrived at the temple at Jerusalem.

There he found Abraham, Moses, and Jesus among the company of prophets. The apostle acted as their *imam* [religious leader] in prayer. Then he was brought two vessels, one containing wine and the other milk. The apostle took the milk and drank it, leaving the wine. Gabriel said: "You have been rightly guided to the way of nature and so will your people be, Muhammad. Wine is forbidden you."

One of Abu Bakrs family told me that "Aysha the prophet's wife used to say: 'The apostle's body remained where it was but God removed his spirit by night.' The apostle described to his companions Abraham, Moses, and Jesus as he saw them that night, saying: "I have never seen a man more like myself than Abraham. Jesus, son of Mary, was a reddish man of medium height with lank hair."

The Night Journey: Meeraj

I heard the apostle say: "After the completion of my business in Jerusalem, a ladder was brought to me finer than any I have ever seen. It was that to which the dying man looks when death approaches. My companion mounted it with me until we came to one of the gates of heaven called the Gate of the Watchers. An angel called Ismail was in charge of it, and under his command were twelve thousand angels." As he told this story, the apostle used to say, "And none knows the armies of God but He." When Gabriel brought me in, Ismail asked who I was, and when he was told that I was Muhammad, he asked if I had been given a mission; and on being assured of this he wished me well.

The apostle told me that the latter said: "All the angels who met me when I entered the lowest heaven smiled in welcome and wished me well, except one who said the same things but did not smile or show that joyful expression which the others had. And when I asked Gabriel the reason, he told me that if he had ever smiled on anyone before or would smile on anyone hereafter he would have smiled on me; but he does not smile because he is Malik, the Keeper of hell. I said to Gabriel "Will you not order him to show me hell?" And he said, "Certainly! O Malik, show Muhammad hell." Thereupon he removed its covering and the flames blazed high into the air until I thought that they would consume everything. So I asked Gabriel to order him to send them back to their place, which he did. I can only compare the effect of their withdrawal to the falling of a shadow, until when the flames retreated whence they had come. Malik placed their cover on them.'

The Apostle said: "When I entered the lowest heaven I saw a man sitting there with the spirits of men passing before him. To one he would speak well and rejoice in him, saying, and 'A good spirit from a good body' and of another he would say 'Faugh' and frown, saying, 'An evil spirit from an evil body.' In answer to my question, Gabriel told me that this was our father Adam, reviewing the spirits of his offspring; the spirit of a believer excited his pleasure, and the spirit of an infidel excited his disgust so that he said the words just quoted.

It is interesting to see that one of the worst punishments is reserved for those who mistreated orphans:

"Then I saw men with lips like camels; in their hands were pieces of fire like stones which they used to thrust into their mouths and they would come out of their posteriors. I was told that these were those who sinfully devoured the wealth of orphans.

The journey continues in hell:

"Then I saw men in the way of the family of Pharaoh, with such bellies as I have never seen; there were passing over them as it were camels maddened by thirst when they were cast into hell, treading them down, they being unable to move out of the way. These were the usurers.
"Then I saw men with good fat meat before them side by side with lean stinking meat, eating the latter and leaving the former. These are those who forsake the women which God has permitted and go after those he has forbidden.
"Then I saw women hanging by their breasts. These were those who had fathered bastards on their husbands." The Apostle said: "Great is God's anger against a woman who brings a bastard into her family. He deprives the true sons of their portion and learns the secrets of the *harim*.
"Then I was taken up to the second heaven and there were two maternal cousins, Jesus, son of Mary, and John, son of Zechariah. Then to the third heaven and there was a man whose face was the moon at the full. This was my brother Joseph, son of Jacob.

The Night Journey: Meeraj

Then to the fourth heaven and there was a man called Idris. 'And we have exalted him to a lofty place.' Then to the fifth heaven, and there was a man with white hair and a long beard; never have I seen a more handsome man than he. This was the beloved among his people Aaron son of 'Imran. Then to the sixth heaven, and there was a dark man with a hooked nose like the Shanu'a. This was my brother Moses, son of Imran. Then to the seventh heaven and there was a man sitting on a throne at the gate of the immortal mansion. Every day seventy thousand angels went in not to come back until resurrection day. Never have I seen a man more like myself. This was my father Abraham. Then he took me into Paradise, and there I saw a damsel with dark red lips and I asked her to whom she belonged, for she pleased me much when I saw her, and she told me 'Zayd b. Hârithah.'" The apostle gave Zayd the good news about her. (Ibn Ishaq, P181–186)

Analysis of The Journey

As a student of psychology, I studied the accepted methods for the interpretation and analysis of dreams, delusions and hallucinations. As a practicing psychologist, I have found that the most practical method for interpretation of dreams is the common sense approach—when examining a given dream within the context of the subject's life experience, pieces will begin to fall into place.

In Muhammad's case, it is known that at the time he had this dream, he was convinced that he was the prophet of Allah. He had amassed a small band of about 100 followers. Although he had many supporters, Muhammad's list of enemies was much longer. He was hated by many and ridiculed mercilessly. What better boost for a prophet under pressure than to have an audience with God Himself? If we accept Carl Jung's theory that the function of dreams is to help create a balance between the conscious and unconscious mind, we can see that this journey clearly provided that balance for Muhammad.

Accompanied by God's personal messenger and riding on the mythical horse of prophets, Muhammad was escorted into the city of prophets: Jerusalem. He was introduced to one prophet after another, eventually culminating in a face to face meeting with the prophet that Muhammad called his "father": Abraham. Muhammad converses with God, surrounded by angels. It is not especially surprising that God justifies Muhammad's anger, blesses his desires, and acknowledges his existential needs. Suddenly, Muhammad's profound feelings of inferiority as a poor orphan are transformed into feelings of grandiosity as he assumes his place as a true prophet of God.

Muhammad's heaven is full of *hurries*: beautiful, heavenly women who are the prizes of heavenly men. Demons torture and burn those who reject Muhammad's message. And who receives the greatest punishment in Muhammad's afterworld? Those who mistreat orphans (a connection could easily be made to Muhammad's childhood deprivations). There are many similar references in the *Quran* to awful consequences of wrong doing to orphans, which demonstrates how bad Muhammad's childhood was and what a strong impact it had on his thinking.

إِنَّ الَّذِينَ يَأْكُلُونَ أَمْوَالَ الْيَتَامَى ظُلْمًا إِنَّمَا يَأْكُلُونَ فِي بُطُونِهِمْ نَارًا وَسَيَصْلَوْنَ سَعِيرًا

[As for] those who swallow the property of the orphans unjustly, surely they only swallow fire into their bellies and they shall enter burning fire. (The *Quran*, 4:10)

Through this dream, Muhammad received complete affirmation of his mission and God's personal confirmation. He received assurance that he was not only favored by God, but also a true prophet on par with Abraham, and that his enemies were God's enemies. No experience could have been as "balancing" and reassuring for a prophet than a journey to heaven. Whether this journey occurred within the context

THE NIGHT JOURNEY: MEERAJ

of a regular dream or was a dream associated with complex partial seizures is of limited significance. What is important is that the experience occurred when Muhammad desperately needed it and that it gave him the strength to continue to live out his mission.

Some of the things that Muhammad sees in heaven are reported in other religions. Although the tour of heaven is only a one-night trip, Muhammad sees many creatures and wonders that would take several lifetimes to observe. Many of these unusual creatures have enormous dimensions and are probably used to emphasize the greatness of God and his heavens. The emphasis on the women of paradise as rewards for men is noted frequently in Islamic literature.

أخبرنا مالك بن إسماعيل أبو غسّان، أخبرنا إسرائيل عن ليث عن مجاهد قال: أعطيَ رسول

الله، صلعم، بُضْع أربعين رجلًا و أعطيَ كلّ رجل من أهل الجنة بُضْع ثمانين

Malik Ibnu Ismail Abu Ghassan reported . . . that Leith heard Mudjahid say: "The Apostle of Allah (PBUH) is endowed with the sexual potency of forty men, and each man of the people of paradise is endowed with that of eighty men." (Ibn Saad 1990, 1:282)

The Prophet often talked about these rewards. He also related to his followers that they were free to drink wine in paradise, a behavior that was totally forbidden in Islam. During the journey, Muhammad fell asleep several times and woke up somewhere else to continue on his voyage. This fact increases the probability that these were several complexes partial seizure dreams. It is interesting to note that the day after the experience; Muhammad decided to let everyone know of his journey and his meeting with God. He expected them to recognize his importance—that he was not just a prophet but also the favorite of them all in the eyes of God and others in paradise. Concerned that the pagans would ridicule him, Muhammad's cousin tried to stop him. But Muhammad was determined to talk about his experience. As it turned out, the cousin was right. Muhammad took so much criticism that he relented and told everyone that he had told them about the dream to determine who the real believers were (rationalization). He used the example of Abraham being told by God to sacrifice his son so that God could see if Abraham would obey Him (intellectualization).

THE INFLUENCE OF ZOROASTRIANISM

One of the earliest Middle Eastern religions to have its own bible was Zoroastrianism. This religion was founded by Zarathustra, or Zartosht, and is so old that nobody knows Zarathushtra's date of birth or death. However, there is general agreement that the religion is older than 800 B.C. and perhaps even as old as 1200 B.C. (Boyce 1995).

Zarathustra was born in a region that today is in the province of Balkh in eastern Afghanistan. He was able to spread his word very quickly. By the time of his death, most of Persia (modern day Iran) was influenced by his teachings.

During the period between A.D 220 to A.D. 700, Christianity and Zoroastrianism were the two dominant religions of the world. The Zoroastrian kings of the Sassanid Dynasty ruled in Iran and the Christian emperors ruled in Rome. However, with the Arab invasion of Iran in the eighth century A.D., the old Persia was gradually drowned in Islam. Eventually, the Iranians developed and incorporated their own sect of Islam called Shiite, which is a combination of Islam and ancient Persian beliefs. In time, the Eastern Roman Empire fell to Islam as well. However, Christianity survived in Europe during the Middle Ages, while the Zoroastrian religion nearly disappeared. Today, there are fewer than 100,000 practicing Zoroastrians in Iran (there are some more in India).

> Zoroastrianism had an enormous influence, directly and indirectly on the history of Christianity and, specifically, of [Christian] hell. These thoughts are based on the early Vedic faith, from which Hinduism and Buddhism also developed,

but instead of relying on pantheon gods, Zoroaster thought a dualistic religion: the divine force of good, Ahuramasda "wise Lord," who lives above with his seven anesha spent ("Immortal holy ones"), he is at war against Evil Spirit "Ahriman," the lord of Lies, who dwells in the darkness of hell under earth, sending out his daevas or devils to torment the world. Law, order and light against darkness filth and death. Their conflict is the history of the world and the object of the conflict is the soul of the man. (Turner 1993, 18)

During a person's life, the archangels in heaven keep track of a person's behavior in two separate accounts, one for good deeds and one for bad. After death, the soul hovers around the head of its corpse for three days while being judged by Rashnu (the genie, or angel of justice and by Mithra (goddess of sun). All good deeds are entered in a great ledger as credits, all wicked actions as debts. At the foot of the underworld Chinvat (Accountant's) Bridge, the reckoning is made. If it is positive, the *Daena*, a beautiful maiden accompanied by two guardian dogs, escorts the soul across the bridge into the House of Song. If negative, "even if the difference is only three tiny acts of wrongdoing," the soul falls into Hell, ruled by Yima (or Yama). If the balance is even, it passes into a kind of limbo called Hammistagan, quite similar to the old Babylonian underworld, where it will stay until the apocalypse. Neither prayer, sacrifice, nor the grace of Ahriman can influence the legal outcome of the mathematical trial.

Eventually, there will be a final cosmic battle between Good and Evil, and Evil will be conquered forever. A savior named Soshyans, born of a virgin impregnated with the seed of Zoroaster, will harrow hell; penitent sinners will be forgiven; and there will be a universal resurrection of the body, which will reunite with the soul. Hell will be destroyed—burned clean by molten metal—and the kingdom of God on earth will begin.... There is an extraordinary similarity between the hells and heavens of Zoroastrianism, Christianity, and Islam. Since Zoroaster was born centuries before Christ, one can postulate that the origin of the fiery hell comes from Zoroastrianism. (Turner 1993)

The term for heaven in Arabic is *Ferdoos,* which is the Arabic form of the Persian and Aramaic word Paradise, meaning "garden" and "heaven."

In Christianity, there are many references to the jaws of hell. The Zoroastrians had their own concept of the jaws of hell centuries earlier; the story is from the Zoroastrian book of *Arda Viraf.* In this story, the hero goes to heaven (which has seven levels) and then passes through hell. Once there, he observes people being tortured by demons in a most gruesome fashion:

> Afterward, Srosh [Messiah] the pious, and Adar [angel of Fire, one of four sacred elements] the angel, took hold of my hand, so that I went on unhurt. In that manner, I beheld cold and heat, drought and stench to such a degree as I never saw, nor have heard, in the world. And when I went farther, I also saw the greedy jaws of hell, like the most frightful pit, descending in a very narrow and fearful Place; in darkness so gloomy that it is necessary to hold by the hand; and in such stench that every one whose nose inhales that air will struggle and stagger and fall (*Arda Viraf* 1:8).

From a historical perspective, the content of the Muhammad's dream of ascension is very similar to the content of the book of *Arda Viraf.* The hero, accompanied by a couple of angels who serve as guides, tours hell and asks questions. One can postulate that these stories were available to Muhammad, just like the stories of Old Testament were. Since Arabs had a great deal of contact with Iranians, Islam was influenced by Zoroastrianism. It appears that both Islam and Christianity incorporated the concepts of heaven and hell found in Zoroastrianism into their faiths, as these concepts do not exist in Judaism. This was a

The Night Journey: Meeraj

useful tool in controlling the crowds and to help put meaning into some aspects of life and death.

One particular similarity between Zoroastrianism and Islam is the punishment for shameless women. In fact, the account in the *Arda Viraf* is almost identical to what Muhammad sees in his tour of hell:

> I also saw the soul of a woman who was suspended, by the breasts, to hell; and its noxious creatures (*khrafstras*) seized her whole body. And I asked thus: "What sin was committed by this body, whose soul suffers such a punishment?" Srosh the pious, and Adar the angel, said thus: "This is the soul of that wicked woman who, in the world, left her own husband, and gave herself to other men, and committed adultery." (*Arda Viraf* 1:7)

Compare this account to a Hadith:

> Having crossed another realm of shadow, the Prophet, mounted on the Buraq and guided by the angel Gabriel, contemplates the sufferings inflicted upon shameless women, particularly those who, by letting their hair be seen by strangers, encouraged criminal relations. The hair hangs up these sinful women, and swirls of flame come from their nostrils. They are guarded by a brown demon with hooked feet, which is wearing ankle-bracelets, breathing fire, and holding a red fork in his hand. "Then I saw women hanging by their breasts. These were those who had fathered bastards on their husbands." (Ibn Ishaq, P186)

Hair is considered one of a woman's principal attractions, and when hidden it is a sign that she is unavailable or has already been chosen. Many places in the *Quran* (see 33:55 and 59; 24:59; and especially 24:31) prescribe that women wear a veil and be modest of demeanor: "Say to the believing women that they must lower their eyes, be chaste, and not display their adornment except what appears thereof. Let their veils cover their breasts! They should not display their adornment except to their husbands, or their fathers" (24:31).

The descriptions of these guilty women and what happens to them in the hells of Zoroastrianism and Islam are too gruesome to describe here. The intention here is only to show the similarities between these religions and demonstrate how the concept of hell came from the Afghan province of Balkh about 3,000 years ago and was then adopted by the religions that came later.

CHAPTER 8

EGO DEFENSES

قُلْ أُوحِيَ إِلَيَّ أَنَّهُ اسْتَمَعَ نَفَرٌ مِّنَ الْجِنِّ فَقَالُوا إِنَّا سَمِعْنَا قُرْآنًا عَجَبًا

Say (O Muhammad SAW): "It has been revealed to me that a group (from three to ten in number) of jinns listened (to this Quran). They said: 'Verily! We have heard a wonderful Recital (this Quran)!'"
—The *Quran*, 72:1

Throughout history, the belief in demons, ghosts, *jinn dives*, and *jinni* has had its own place. However, with time and education (mainly through the methods of mass communication), these beliefs have lost their value and importance and have become superstitions. Although many people and religions still hang on to these imaginary creatures, they do not hold any place in science except as part of a study on mythology and human cultural history.

The origins of these metaphysical creatures are lost in human history, but they are perhaps related to the fears that humans suffered during prehistoric centuries. In English there are many names for these beings; however, in Middle Eastern languages, one word has a special and universal meaning for all Moslems: *jinn*. There are frequent references to *jinns* in the *Quran*—in fact, there is a 28-verse *sura* entirely about *jinns*.

Muhammad fought against the common superstitions of the time, but his frequent references to *jinns* has given ammunition to his critics to ridicule him or to use as proof that he had paranoid tendencies. However, the intention here is not to use the story of Muhammad and the *jinns* to ridicule him. This story, like others in his life, is useful for understanding the psychodynamics of Muhammad's inter psychic forces and further validating the hypotheses of his illness.

THE YEAR OF DEPRESSION

The tenth year after Muhammad's claim to be Prophet of Islam was one of the worst years of his life. The events of this year were so bad that he called it the "Year of Sadness." He had been a self-proclaimed prophet for 10 years, but things were not going his way. He had only about 100 followers. One group had immigrated to Ethiopia to avoid the pressures of the pagans, and those living in Mecca were also having a difficult time.

MUHAMMAD'S TROUBLES

Muhammad was lucky to have the protection of his clan under the name of his uncle Abu Taleb, who had raised him. But the pagans (the tribe of Ghouraish) put severe sanctions on Muhammad and his followers, and they were poor and badly restricted. Muhammad's followers were dissatisfied with the lack of improvement in their conditions. Then there was the sudden death of Muhammad's beloved wife Khadijeh—her death was quite hard on him.

Khadijeh had provided Muhammad's main psychological support, and it was her wealth that had turned things around for him. She was the first Moslem, and it was she who had assured him that he was not going crazy. She was the first woman in his life, and he never betrayed her by taking additional wives during her lifetime (as was common for Arab men at that time). Most important of all, Khadijeh was the mother figure that he never had.

Ego Defenses

Within two months, Muhammad's uncle, Abu Taleb, died as well. The old man's protection had been the only reason Muhammad was still alive. Without his uncle, there was no reason for the pagans not to kill him.

One day on his way home, a woman threw the genitals and womb of a goat at him. Still, the pagans were not ready to kill him and start a clan war. His followers, however (who were mostly commoners of lower status) were fair game for their assaults. Torture was commonplace. This angered his followers—after all, if Muhammad had such a close affiliation with God, why couldn't he provide any support for them? Some of the followers renounced Islam and went back to their old religions to avoid hardship and death.

Muhammad's Journey to Taief

The Prophet was badly depressed and needed a way out. The best solution would have been to immigrate to a new city, but no one dared to give him sanctuary and risk the wrath of the pagans. However, about 100 miles outside of Mecca, there was a famous city called Taief. The city was located on higher elevations, so it had water and a cooler climate (today, it is a resort city for the Saudi royal family). Since the city had water, it also supported agriculture (mostly grapes). The tribe living in Taief was the Bani Thagif, a rich and powerful tribe that Muhammad believed could potentially stand up against the people of Mecca. So, Muhammad decided to try his luck to see if the Bani Thagif would be willing to give him sanctuary.

Muhammad traveled alone on his journey to Taief, but to his surprise, he discovered that the people of the city were not receptive to him at all. They did not want to risk irritating the Ghouraish, so they completely rejected him. Muhammad asked the people of Taief to at least not tell the people of Mecca about his trip there, as he was concerned that the pagans would get even angrier with him. But they rejected that too, saying that the people of Mecca would eventually know and that if they didn't reveal that information, there would be hell to pay. The Bani Thagif not only rejected Muhammad, but also chased him out of the city. The children threw stones at him as he left, one of which hit his leg and caused him to bleed. Muhammad ran into a vineyard and hid, where he was reportedly saved by a slave. The road back home was long, so he stopped in a village for the night.

THE STORY OF THE SEVEN JINNS

The place that Muhammad stayed for the night was a village called Nakhleh. It had been called "the village of *jinns*" as well (Makarem Shirazi 1995, 100), which indicates that there must have been some connection between the village and stories about demons in the past. That night, Muhammad spent some time praying and reciting the *Quran*.

As the story goes, seven *jinns* were also staying in Nakhleh over night on their way from Yemen (Al-Tabari, Persian translation, 1990, 3:889). They heard the words of the *Quran* and were mesmerized by it, so they became Moslems and took the word to their city. Since many of them converted to Islam, the *jinns* became divided into two groups: believers and nonbelievers. Satan is believed to be non-believing *jinn* (Ayatollah Makarem Shirazi 1995, 25:100 –140).

قُلْ أُوحِيَ إِلَيَّ أَنَّهُ اسْتَمَعَ نَفَرٌ مِّنَ الْجِنِّ فَقَالُوا إِنَّا سَمِعْنَا قُرْآنًا عَجَبًا

Say: It has been revealed to me that a party of the jinn listened, and they said: "Surely we have heard a wonderful Quran,

يَهْدِي إِلَى الرُّشْدِ فَآمَنَّا بِهِ وَلَن نُّشْرِكَ بِرَبِّنَا أَحَدًا

Guiding to the right way, so we believe in it, and we will not set up any one with our Lord.

وَأَنَّهُ تَعَالَى جَدُّ رَبِّنَا مَا اتَّخَذَ صَاحِبَةً وَلَا وَلَدًا

And that He—exalted be the majesty of our Lord—has not taken a consort, nor a son." (The Quran, 72:1–3)

Analysis of Muhammad's Ego Defenses

Although this story could be easily rejected as Muhammad's superstition, the fact that it is written in the *Quran* makes it a fact in Islam that a Moslem can not reject as nonexistent. (I remember once when I asked a teacher of religious studies in high school about the validity of *jinns*, he simply answered that we are Moslems—it is written in the *Quran*, so we believe in it.)

This story has been interpreted by researchers not friendly to Islam in many different ways, but these researchers usually try to use it to discredit Muhammad. However, the story does provide some valuable information regarding Muhammad's mind, especially concerning his ego defense mechanisms. Given the stress that Muhammad was experiencing at the time—he had lost an important loved one, his religion was stagnating, the people of Taief had thrown stones at him, and even his followers were renouncing him—it is interesting to note that Muhammad was suddenly accepted by *jinns*. In effect, the story of the seven *jinns* indicates that Muhammad's primary ego defense mechanisms are compensation and rationalization.

"Compensation" refers to a defense mechanism that is "operating unconsciously, by which one attempts to make up for real or fancied deficiencies. It also refers to a conscious process in which one strives to make up for real or imagined defects of physique, performance skills, or psychological attributes. The two types frequently merge" (Abess 2003). In Muhammad's case, the rationale behind the story of the *jinns* was to compensate for rejection. In Muhammad's mind, if human beings rejected him, so be it—there were other creatures of God (the *jinns*) who would accept him.

Rationalization was also one of Muhammad's primary ego defenses. Actually, one way or another, most of Muhammad's behaviors were rationalizations. Rationalization refers to "common-sense, utilitarian justifications of internal and external conditions. It is an effort to justify attitudes, beliefs, or behaviors that are irrational or otherwise unacceptable by the arbitrary application of a truth—a so called 'logical explanation'—or by the invention of a convincing fallacy. Rationalization is the unconsciously motivated and involuntary act of giving logical and believable explanations for irrational behaviors that have been prompted by unacceptable, unconscious wishes, or by the defenses used to cope with such wishes" (Valliant 1986).

The story of the seven *jinns* is certainly related to rationalization, but there are numerous other examples as well. One of the most famous events in which Muhammad used rationalization is when he gave too much to the leaders of Ghouraish after the conquest of the Hawazan. The Ghouraish received a great deal of loot and wealth, and Muhammad's followers were angry that he had given the camels and silver to the old enemies of Islam (the Ghouraish were pagans who had made life miserable for Muhammad and his followers before they were converted to Islam by force). Muhammad made a speech to his followers, telling them that while it was true the Ghouraish had the wealth, silver, and camels, they had God's Prophet.

> When the apostle had distributed the gifts among Ghouraish and the Bedouin tribes, and the Ansar got nothing, this tribe of Ansar took the matter to heart and talked a great deal about it, until one of them said, "By God, the apostle has met his own people." Saad b. 'Ubada went to the apostle and told him what had happened. He asked, "Where do you stand in this matter, Saad?" He said, "I stand with my people." "Then gather your people in this enclosure," he said. He did so, and when some of the Muhajirs came, he let them come, while others he sent back. When he had got them altogether he went and told the apostle and he came to them, and after praising and thanking God he addressed them thus: "O men of Ansar, what is this I hear of you? Do you think ill of me in your hearts? Did I not come to you when you were erring and God guided you; poor and God made you rich; enemies and God softened your hearts?"

They answered; "Yes indeed, God and his Apostle are most kind and generous." He continued: "Why don't you answer me. O Ansar?" They said, "How shall we answer you? Kindness and generosity belong to God and His apostle." He said, "Had you so wished you could have said—and you would have spoken the truth and have been believed—you came to us discredited and we believed you; deserted and we helped you; a fugitive and we took you in; poor and we comforted you. Are you disturbed in mind because of the good things of this life by which I win over a people that they may become Muslims while I entrust you to your Islam? Are you not satisfied that men should take away flocks and herds while you take back with you the apostle of God? By him in whose hand is the soul of Muhammad, but the migration I should be one of the Ansar myself. If all men went one way and the Ansar another I should take the way of the Ansar. God have mercy on the Ansar, their sons and their sons' sons." The people wept until the tears ran down their beards as they said, "We are satisfied with the apostle of God as our lot and portion." Then the apostle went off and they dispersed." (Ibn Ishaq, P 596–597)

This clever speech that got Muhammad out of the political jam is an excellent use of rationalization. He had given the loot to Ghouraish for personal reasons—to show off to people who had put him down throughout the years, to create unity among different tribes, and to ease up tensions between old enemies—but he did not include any of these reasons in his answer to his followers. Instead, he merely tried to make his followers feel better by telling them that regardless of the wealth that the Ghouraish had been allowed to retain, they had been given the greater privilege of being in the presence of the prophet of God.

CHAPTER 9

THE DEATH OF THE PROPHET

O people of the graves! Happy are you that you are so much better off than men here

—Muhammad

MUHAMMAD'S FINAL VICTORIES

In the sixth year after his migration to Medina, the Prophet decided to perform the pilgrimage to Mecca, something that had been denied to the Muslims by the pagans. Fourteen hundred of the Prophet's followers volunteered to accompany him. Muhammad directed the Muslims not to carry any arms other than swords—a weapon of travelers, not warriors. Moslems camped at Hudaibiyah, 10 miles from Mecca.

An envoy was sent to the pagans of Mecca to obtain permission for visiting the Kaaba, but the pagans sent their envoy to tell the Prophet that he was not allowed. The Prophet stated that he had not gone there to fight but to perform the pilgrimage. The pagans refused Muhammad entry into Mecca altogether. After much negotiation, however, a treaty was drafted to permit the Moslems to come back the following year; also, they signed a peace agreement for 10 years.

Sword And Seizure

Muhammad's friends were furious with him, for they did not want to accept this disrespect. However, this peace treaty, known as Hudaibiyah, turned out to be one of the most fruitful political moves of Muhammad's life. The 10-year peace allowed him to bring his message to all the people of Arabia and destroy the rest of his enemies (Al-Tabari, Persian translation, 1990, 4:1110).

Victory Over Khaibar

Upon his return to Medina, Muhammad had to come up with a victory to appease his angry followers and as usual the Jewish tribes were the best target, as they would provide the most treasure to loot. The Prophet began preparation for an attack on the Jewish fortifications of Khaibar. In August of A.D. 628, his army of 1,600 well-equipped soldiers left Medina for Khaibar. The force was empowered with 200 horseman, giving Muhammad a great advantage that he did not have in previous battles. Khaibar was a rich oasis and home to the remainder of the Jewish tribes of Arabia. They owned fertile land and the wealth of generations of commerce. Muhammad executed his plans so well that the people of Khaibar were taken by total surprise, and with some heroic efforts by his followers, he was able to open the fortresses one by one. Finally, Muhammad reached the last of the castles where his cousin, Ali, was able to break through the gates in a historic fight and win the war for the Prophet.

Muhammad tortured and then killed the leader of the Jews, Kananeh, and took his 17-year-old wife, Safieh, as his own. He took his own 20 percent of the booty and gave the rest to his followers. This type of success on the battlefield in Arabia brought with it a kind of admiration to Muhammad beyond recognition.

Victory Over the Pagans

One of the conditions of the treaty of Hudaibiyah was that the pagans would not be allowed to fight against any ally of the Muslims, nor would

THE DEATH OF THE PROPHET

the Muslims be permitted to fight against any ally of the pagans. In simple language, the clause of the cease-fire included the allies as well as the principals. However, eight years after Muhammad's migration to Medina, one of the Moslem allies was attacked by pagan allies. The treaty was broken and the deal was off, but by that time Muhammad's army had grown so large that he no longer needed to fear any enemy.

The time had come to free Mecca from the pagans and all other enemies of Islam. The Prophet marched with 10,000 men on the tenth of Ramadan (A.D..630) and camped a short distance from Mecca. The pagan chief, Abu Sufyan, had to give in, and the next day the Muslim army triumphantly marched into Mecca.

The people of Mecca had scoffed and jeered at Muhammad's prophetic mission, ruthlessly persecuted him and his disciples, and ultimately drove them away, creating all manner of obstacles to the propagation of the faith and waging war upon war on the Muslims. This same city now lay at Muhammad's feet. At this moment of triumph, he could have done anything he wished with the city and the citizens. However, he had not come for revenge. He ordered only six people to be killed who had ridiculed his prophesy in his absence, and forgave everybody else.

Finally, Muhammad was able to do what Abraham had done—destroy all of the idols of the Kaaba. Entering the Kaaba, the Prophet began breaking and demolishing the idols. There were 360 idols fixed with lead or tin in the walls and on the roof. To every idol that the Prophet went toward, he would point his cane and say:

وَقُلْ جَاءَ الْحَقُّ وَزَهَقَ الْبَاطِلُ إِنَّ الْبَاطِلَ كَانَ زَهُوقًا

The truth has come and the falsehood has vanished; surely falsehood is destined to vanish. (The *Quran*, 17:81)

Having dwelt upon the equality and brotherhood of mankind and preaching the unity and omnipotence of God, he inquired from the pagans. They asked for kindness and pity, The Prophet recited a few verses of the Quran and forgave every one, including his most staunch enemy,

Abu Sufian (Ibn Ishaq, 553).

قَالَ لَا تَثْرِيبَ عَلَيْكُمُ الْيَوْمَ يَغْفِرُ اللَّهُ لَكُمْ وَهُوَ أَرْحَمُ الرَّاحِمِينَ

He said: (There shall be) no reproof against you this day; Allah may forgive you, and He is the most Merciful of the merciful. (The Quran, 12:9)

The result of this magnanimity and compassion was that those diehards who had relentlessly opposed the Prophet and refused to listen to his message converged around him in their multitudes and accepted Islam. Once the people of Mecca submitted to the faith, disciples were sent out to all neighboring tribes to invite them, with peace and goodwill, to embrace Islam. Many tribes responded to the call.

THE LAST SERMON

The ninth and tenth years of Muhammad's life in Medina were quite fruitful. Although there were many battles, Muhammad was able to win them all and get his message to all of Arabia and beyond. In his eleventh year in Medina, Muhammad made a final pilgrimage to Mecca at the age of 63. Feeling that the end was close, Muhammad made a famous speech to emphasize several points of his teachings He praised and glorified God, and then he said:

> O men, listen to my words. I do not know whether I shall ever meet you in this place again after this year. Your blood and your property are sacrosanct until you meet your Lord, as this day and this month are holy. You will surely meet your Lord and He will ask you of your works. I have told you. He, who has a pledge, let him return it to him who entrusted him with it; all usury is

abolished, but you have your capital. Wrong not and you shall not be wronged. God has decreed that there is to be no usury and the usury of 'Abbas b. 'Abdul-Muttalib is abolished, all of it. All blood shed in the pagan period is to be left Unavenged. The first claim on blood I abolish is that of Rabiab. Al-Harith b, Abdul-Muttalib (who was fostered among the B. Layth and whom Hudhayl killed) it is the first bloodshed in the pagan period, which I deal with. Satan despairs of ever being worshipped in your land, but if he can be obeyed in anything short of worship he will be pleased in matters you may be disposed to think of little account, so beware of him in your religion. Postponement of a sacred month is only an excess of disbelief whereby those who disbelieve are misled; they allow it one year and forbid it another year that they may make up the number of months which God has allowed, so that they permit what God has forbidden, and forbid what God has allowed. Time has completed its cycle and is as it was on the day that God created the heavens and the earth. The number of months with God is twelve; four of them are sacred, three consecutive and the Rajab of Mudar, which is between Jumada and Shaban.

You have rights over your wives and they have rights over you. You have the right that they should not defile your bed and that they should not behave with open unseemliness. If they do, God allows you to put them in separate rooms and to beat them, but not with severity. If they refrain from these things they have the right to their food and clothing with kindness. Lay injunctions on women kindly, for they are prisoners with you having no control of their persons. You have taken them only as a trust from God, and you have the enjoyment of their persons by the words of God, so understand (and listen to) my words, O men, for I have told you. I have left with you something which if you will hold fast to it you will never fall into error—a plain indication, the book of God and the practice of His prophet, so give good heed to what I say.

Know that every Muslim is a Muslim's brother, and that the Muslims are brethren. It is only lawful to take from a brother what he gives you willingly, so wrong not yourselves. O God, have I not told you?

I was told that the men said "O God, yes," and the apostle said "O God, bear witness." Then the apostle continued his pilgrimage and showed the men the rites and taught them the customs of their *hajj*. (Ibn Ishaq, 651–652)

Why did Muhammad feel the need to give this final sermon? Until that time, he had dealt with Arabs in small groups. He finally had representation from all the tribes and clans to make his points. Many years had past since he began his ministry, so he now needed to clarify and emphasize several issues.

Muhammad considered unifying the Arabs to be one of the most important aspects of his mission. He knew that if the Arabs were united, they could take Islam to other lands; but if they continued the old tribal feuds, Islam would be isolated to Arabia. This was the reason why he took the opportunity to put an end to all blood grievances of pre-Islam and create a new beginning in which those feuds were null and void. In addition, at a personal level, he wanted to finish his mission with God. He looked at the skies several times, taking God as a witness that he did what he was supposed to do. He wanted God and all people surrounding him to know that he had done his job.

LAST SERMON, AND THE FAITH OF THE WOMEN

Muhammad's relationship with his mother and his wives was reported in previous chapters. However, his rulings on the topic of women's rights have had profound impact on the lives of millions of Moslem women

THE DEATH OF THE PROPHET

throughout history. Muhammad's teachings were progressive for his time and place. However, the concrete and straightforward manner in which these teachings were presented has created many current problems in the Middle East.

Before Muhammad, women of Arabia had very limited rights. They were not considered much more than cattle. Muhammad—perhaps because of his own kindness towards the weak, his psychological dependency on women, and the loss of his mother at a young age—came up with some rules that increased the status of women in his society. He limited the number of wives that a man could have to four, set strict standards for inheritance, and protected the financial rights of women. His respectful manner of dealing with his nanny and wives set the precedent to respect older women and family members. However, when applied to today's societies, these standards simply fall short and in many instances could be considered cruel.

Muhammad's rulings regarding women are clearly spelled out in the fourth *sura* of the *Quran*. However, one of the verses in this *sura* (as well as portions of Muhammad's last sermon) has provided men in Moslem societies with the opportunity to oppress women.

The portion of the *Quran* concerning this issue is:

الرِّجَالُ قَوَّامُونَ عَلَى النِّسَاءِ بِمَا فَضَّلَ اللهُ بَعْضَهُمْ عَلَى بَعْضٍ وَبِمَا أَنْفَقُوا مِنْ أَمْوَالِهِمْ فَالصَّالِحَاتُ قَانِتَاتٌ حَافِظَاتٌ لِلْغَيْبِ بِمَا حَفِظَ اللهُ وَاللَّاتِي تَخَافُونَ نُشُوزَهُنَّ فَعِظُوهُنَّ وَاهْجُرُوهُنَّ فِي الْمَضَاجِعِ وَاضْرِبُوهُنَّ فَإِنْ أَطَعْنَكُمْ فَلَا تَبْغُوا عَلَيْهِنَّ سَبِيلًا إِنَّ اللهَ كَانَ عَلِيًّا كَبِيرًا

Men are in charge of women because Allah has made some of them to excel others and because they spend out of their property; the good women are therefore obedient, guarding the unseen as Allah has guarded; and [as to] those on whose part you fear desertion, admonish them, and leave them alone in the sleeping-places and beat them; then if they obey you, do not seek away against them; surely Allah is high, great. (4:34)

The first few words of this verse have been translated into English differently by different translators (Shakir, Yusuf Ali), but the traditional translation and its true meaning is that "men are in charge of women." Men are considered to be the head of the family, its ruler, and its protector. Therefore, if a woman does not obey the husband, the man can admonish her, distance himself from her, or deprive her from sex—and if this doesn't work, he can then beat her.

Considering Muhammad's power, one can postulate that if he simply had forbidden physical punishment of women, life would have been much easier for them. Many of the interpreters of the *Quran* have referred to physical punishment as last resort, but there are no real standards on the extent and severity of beatings. It appears that as long as the ones administering the beatings do not break any bones, they can not be taken to Islamic court.

The interpreters of the *Quran* have come up with different rationalizations for this cruel ruling, some of which are simply astonishing. Ayatollah Makarem Shirazi, who is currently among the ruling class in Iran, wrote the following:

> Today's psychoanalysts believe that a group of women have a condition called "masochism." And sometimes, when this condition gets really strong, the only method of settling it down is light physical punishment. Therefore, in such cases, light physical punishment is a form of psychotherapy. (Ayatollah Makarem Shirazi 1995, 3:373–374)

THE PROPHET'S ILLNESS

During his eleventh year in Medina, Muhammad developed the illness that would eventually take his life. A glance at his symptoms clearly shows that he died of some kind of neurological problem. Since hundreds of people witnessed these events, the reports are very similar.

The beginning of the end started when the Prophet called his servant to go with him to the cemetery of Baqi in the middle of the night. Once he arrived there, he prayed for all those who had been killed in previous battles, saying:

> Peace upon you, O people of the graves! Happy are you that you are so much better off than men here. Dissensions have come like waves of darkness one after the other, the last being worse than the first. (Ibn Ishaq, 678)

Muhammad was bothered by the dissention among his followers, who were juggling for leadership after his imminent death. Muhammad told his friends that "I have been given the choice between the keys of the treasuries of this world and long life here, followed by Paradise, and meeting my Lord and Paradise at once" (Ibn Ishaq, 678). Muhammad left the cemetery and went home, and in the morning his illness began. The Prophet's wife Aysha said:

> The Apostle returned from the cemetery to find me suffering a severe headache, and I was saying, "O my head!" He said, "Nay, 'Aysha, "O my head!" Then he said, "Would it distress you if you were to die before me so that I might wrap you in your shroud and pray over you and bury you?" I said, "I see if you had done that returning to my house and spending a bridal night with one of your wives." The Apostle smiled, and then his pain overcame him as he was going the round of his wives, until he was overpowered in the house of Maymuna. He called his wives and asked their permission to be nursed in my house, and they agreed. (Ibn Ishaq, P679)

Sword And Seizure

The Apostle went out walking, helped by Abbas and Ali, his head bound in a cloth and his feet dragging. "Then the Apostle's illness worsened and he suffered much pain. He said, 'Pour seven skins of water from different wells over me so that I may go out to the men and instruct them.' His wives made him sit down in a tub and poured water over him until he cried, "Enough, enough!" (Ibn Ishaq, P679).

Muhammad then went to the mosque for prayers and to let his followers know that the end had come. When he came back home, his pain increased until he was exhausted. Some of his wives gathered to him with some family members, and they agreed to force him to take medicine. He soon recovered, after which he became angry with his family for giving him medicine. He told all of them to take the same medicine that he had been given as punishment for what they had done to him.

When the Prophet's condition worsened, he ordered the people to tell Abu Bakr to superintend the prayers. Muhammad was, however, able to make it to morning prayers, and when the Muslims saw him, they were almost seduced from their prayers for joy at seeing him. But Muhammad motioned to them that they should continue. The Apostle smiled with joy when he saw Moslems in prayer. Ayesha relates:

> The Apostle came back to me from the mosque that day and lay in my bosom. A man of Abu Bakr's family came in to me with a toothpick in his hand and the apostle looked at it in such a way that I knew he wanted it, and when I asked him if he wanted me to give it to him he said yes; so I took it and chewed it for him to soften it and gave it to him. He rubbed his teeth with it more energetically than I had ever seen him rub before; then he laid it down. I found him heavy in my bosom and as I looked into his face, his eyes were fixed. (Ibn Ishaq, P682)

Muhammad's symptoms during his final days—his severe head ache and dragging his feet, his inability to talk (Ibn Ishaq, P 680) and communicating with nodding, his vigorous use of a toothbrush (Ibn Saad

The Death of the Prophet

1990, 180), and his hallucinations (Al-Tabari 1990, 4:1320)—all point to high likelihood that he died of the seizures (perhaps accompanied by a stroke).

Muhammad died on June 8, A.D. 632, in Medina. Using his teachings and methods, his followers conquered all the lands from China to Spain. Today, Moslems dominate most of Asia and Africa. Although, like other religions, Moslems are divided into many different groups, the existence of the *Quran* has kept the foundations of the religion of Islam unified throughout the history.

Muhammad's accomplishments make him one of the most influential men in human history. However, his claim of being a messenger of God is simply a byproduct of his seizure disorder—nothing more and nothing less.

APPENDIX I

COMPLEX PARTIAL SEIZURES

Although schizophrenia and complex partial seizures are two entirely different conditions, there is an inherent correlation between the two diseases. It appears that these two conditions are heavily interrelated due to their involvement with the left temporal lobes. Those suffering from seizure disorder (also known as epileptics) make appearances in the Bible and in other ancient texts, some dating back 4,000 years. Alexander of Macedonia, Joan of Arc and the Russian novelist Dostoyevsky are all said to have suffered from seizures (Savor 1997, Geschwind 1983). It is not surprising then that epilepsy, in its various manifestations, has been studied extensively since the earliest stages of human civilization

EPILEPSY (SEIZURE DISORDER)

The fascination with epilepsy is as old as the disease itself. Like many other phenomena in ancient society, if people did not understand the cause of something, they often declared it to be the work of the gods. When the ancient Greeks observed men being grabbed by something, falling down, and then getting squeezed as if their life was coming out of them, they thought that gods must have seized that person and thrown him or her to the ground. This is where the term "seizure" originates. Since it was believed that the gods seized a person, the condition was sometimes also referred to as the "Sacred Disease" or the "Falling Disease" (Moore 1997).

Ancient Greek physicians were the first to try and bring some kind of logic to this condition. Hippocrates, the father of medicine, wrote of epilepsy and its relationship to the brain. Galen, the Roman Imperial physician, investigated this condition in a better light and brought the illness down from the skies and the gods and classified it as a real disease. Galen noticed that his epileptic patients often complained of odd sensations prior to their seizures. One patient described it as a mysterious cool breeze. Galen labeled the phenomenon aura, the Latin word for breeze or wind. The aura is considered the initial prelude to the devastating symptoms of the disease that occur shortly thereafter.

Many early physicians noticed that some children with epilepsy grew out of it when they reached puberty. They therefore concluded that sexual acts were the cure. In order to get the children to grow up more quickly sexually, physicians subjected them to horrible sexual behaviors. It was only during the second century B.C. that a Greek physician named Aretaeus rejected these primitive methods, suggesting that the process of growth has its own time line and that the cure had to be found elsewhere (Adams 1856).

Unfortunately, Aretaeus's remedies were not much more advanced than his predecessors—he suggested inserting medicine into the mouth of patients while they were unconscious (this is now completely rejected, as it can cause suffocation). Inserting similar medications into rectums of younger patients, bloodletting, and other primitive treatments were also commonplace. However, Aretaeus eventually came up with a diagnosis known as "interictal personality disorder," which is the idea that patients with intractable epilepsy eventually tend to develop a host of other symptoms that seem to have little to do with the seizures, and nothing to do with the supernatural. Aretaeus was able to document that there is a high prevalence of depression among patients suffering

Appendix I: Complex Partial Seizures

from epilepsy. However, he thought that all of these symptoms stemmed from the shame surrounding the patient's inability to control his or her body.

The Dark Ages were very dark indeed when it came to dealing with diseases, and no real progress was made toward further diagnosing or curing the disease. Most likely, epileptics were punished and whipped with a lash in the same manner that psychiatric patients were in order to get the demons out of them. Thankfully, the thirteenth and fourteenth centuries brought a revival of science. This period was the beginning of exploration into the disease in a more logical fashion. The methods of learning about the disease changed to documenting and working on the symptoms.

By the seventeenth and eighteenth centuries, the concept of demons and gods as the source of the disease was totally rejected. Epilepsy was considered to be a natural disease. The advent of newer hospitals equipped with better staff, teachers, and students provided the opportunity to hospitalize patients and explore their diseases in a more systematic fashion. "Early psychiatrists like Faliet and Morel, and English neurologists like Prichard and Russell were among the first to study epilepsy with a view toward determining its true pathology. But it would be another two hundred years before scientists could clearly explain the origins of the mysterious condition" (Moore 1997).

During the nineteenth century, a new problem arose when histrionic women, imitating the Victorian Era collapses, began pretending to suffer from epilepsy and filled the psychiatric hospitals. For the new world of scientists trying to better understand seizure disorder, this was a setback—but only a temporary one. Noted psychoanalysts such as Freud and his followers were able to make the proper differential diagnosis between hysteria and true seizures.

> In 1845, a French doctor named Esquire studied 349 epileptic women housed in a hospital seizure ward. He attempted to focus on the difference between 46 so-called "hysterical" patients and

the epileptic patients. On the surface, their symptoms were so similar that hysteria and epilepsy were often confused with each other. But the epileptic patients were unique. Another researcher, Faliet, focused his efforts on defining this interictal pathology of epilepsy. He believed epilepsy to be a cerebral condition leading to all sorts of secondary mental disorders. Faliet's description of post-ictal psychosis is remarkably similar to the modern concept. Like Aretaeus centuries before, Faliet also advanced the concept of Interictal Personality Disorder or "epileptic character." Morel, writing in 1816, put forth the same idea but went a step further to define what he called "masked" epilepsy. This, Morel explained, was a more subtle form of epilepsy in which seizures lacked convulsive activity but presented, instead, with disturbances in thought and behavior. (Moore 1997)

Neurons and The Brain

In order to be able to understand the mechanism of an epileptic attack, it is important to first have a basic familiarity with a brain cell, or neuron. A typical neuron, is made of three different parts. These include (1) the body of the cell, which includes the nuclei and is the center of life for the cell; (2) an axon, which is the long tube coming out of the cell that is in charge of transmitting information from one cell to the other one; and (3) the dendrites, which are the branches at the different corners of the cell that connect one cell to the other. The tubular is comprised of:

> An inner section and an outer cell wall or membrane. The chemical composition of the inside of a nerve cell is very different from that of the outside. Specifically, there is a difference in the concentration of sodium and potassium salts. Sodium concentration is highest on the outside of the cell while potassium dominates inside. In the cell's normal resting state, a series of membrane pumps are constantly working to maintain the proper balance of these salts.

Appendix I: Complex Partial Seizures

When a nerve is called upon to transmit an electrical signal, there is a sudden movement of these salts from one side of the cell membrane to the other. This movement spreads like a wave from one end of the nerve to the other until it reaches the end. At this point, the nerve's signal may be transmitted to the next nerve cell either by a direct extension of this process or, more commonly, by releasing a chemical called a neurotransmitter. Neurotransmitters fall into one of two categories. The "excitatory" neurotransmitters are responsible for facilitating cell-to-cell communication while "inhibitory" neurotransmitters serve to slow down or even stop cell-to-cell communication. Over activity of excitatory neurotransmitters or under activity of inhibitory neurotransmitters results in an uncoordinated flow of electrical activity in the brain and can, in some cases, trigger seizures. (Lishman 1997)

Human brain is divided into two hemispheres, each hemisphere includes: frontal lobe, parietal lobe, occipital lobe and the temporal lobe. The temporal lobe is located near the temples. Like other parts of brain, the temporal lobes are involved in conducting many different tasks. It has been widely accepted that the temporal lobes serve an important function in language processes. Specifically, it is known that the left temporal lobe plays a significant role in how humans comprehend spoken language. It is also believed that the temporal lobes are involved in some of the complex aspects of vision, including the ability to perceive patterns, such as faces.

The temporal lobes are also involved in emotional aspects of human life. The left temporal lobe is highly critical in verbal memory. The lower parts of the temporal lobes are the seat for most nouns, while the parts closer to the movement strip of frontal lobes are more the seats for verbs. Right-sided lesions result in impairment of recall of nonverbal material, such as music and drawings. Temporal lobes help in sorting new information and are believed to be responsible for short-term memory. The right temporal lobe is mainly involved in visual memory (i.e. memory for pictures and faces). The temporal lobes are involved in the primary organization and sequencing of sensory input (Read 1981).

STAGES OF SEIZURES

Epilepsy is usually a chronic condition that is characterized by frequent abnormal electrical discharges from brain cells. These attacks typically originate in the cerebral cortex. Epilepsy is either "symptomatic," meaning secondary to a particular brain abnormality, or "idiopathic," meaning without a clear cause. In a normal brain, the nerve transmissions are regular and quite complex. But during a seizure, these neurons generate uncoordinated electrical discharges that spread throughout the brain and create a domino effect that leads to severe changes in the person's behavior. These changes can occur with both normal and abnormal nerve cells (Engel 1996).

Seizures are typically divided into three distinct parts: (1) the aura, which is a period of warning prior to a seizure during which patients sometimes feel strange physical sensations, experience visual abnormalities, or detect unusual smells; (2) the seizure itself, which is known as the ictus; and (3) the postictal state, which is the period of time immediately following the seizure.

Seizures most often begin in one of two areas of the brain: the motor cortex (which is responsible for the initiation of body movement) or the temporal lobes (which include a deep area called the hippocampus that is involved in memory). Nerve cells in these areas appear to be particularly sensitive to situations that can provoke abnormal electrical transmission. Such situations might include decreased oxygen level, metabolic changes, or infection. In some people, any one of these situations can trigger a seizure.

Many types of problems or abnormalities can trigger a seizure. Once the process has started, it follows a course that is specific for each individual person. The local problem can quickly spread to other parts of

Appendix I: Complex Partial Seizures

the brain and create the symptoms listed above. If seizure activity runs for more than 20 minutes, it can also further damage the area of the brain in which it takes place, or even damage other areas of the brain. Frequent uncontrolled seizures without medical care are a dangerous condition that can result in death.

Types of Seizures

In United States alone, four million people suffer from epilepsy, which shows just how common this condition is. The image that most people have of a seizure is one of a person falling to the ground in convulsions, foaming at the mouth, biting his or her tongue, and having no memory of the episode when it is over. While this is characteristic of one type of seizure (grand mal), there are many other types.

A seizure can be broadly defined as an involuntary symptom or behavior that is due to abnormal electrical activity in the brain. Seizures may result in dramatic movements, unusual sensations, or even alterations in consciousness. Despite the wide variety of possible seizure symptoms, most seizures fall into one of just a few general categories. To begin with, a seizure is first classified as either generalized or partial (Engel 1996).

Generalized Seizures

Generalized seizures are caused by abnormal electrical activity and occur over the entire brain simultaneously. This group of seizures affects the level of the patient's awareness and muscle movement of all his or her extremities. The type of generalized seizure that most people think of when discussing epilepsy is called the grand mal or tonic-clonic seizure.

A person experiencing a tonic-clonic seizure typically collapses, stiffens (becomes tonic), and begins rhythmic muscular jerking (becomes clonic). The patient's breathing is shallow during the seizure and the lack of oxygen causes the color of his or her skin to change. The person typically drools and experiences a loss of bowel and bladder control.

Grand mal seizures usually last a couple of minutes, after which time normal breathing and consciousness returns. Patients usually suffer from fatigue after the seizure is over. Since there is no aura prior to a grand mal seizure, there is no warning for the patient, and he or she is usually badly taken off guard.

In addition to grand mal or tonic-clonic type seizure, there are four other types of generalized seizures: absence seizures, myoclonic seizures, tonic seizures, and atonic seizures. Absence seizures are a relatively mild type of seizure that causes unconsciousness without convulsions. They are typically short, usually lasting only 2 to 10 seconds. An absence seizure begins abruptly and without warning, consists of a period of unconsciousness in which the patient exudes a blank stare, and then ends abruptly. After the seizure, the patient is usually unaware that anything has happened. He or she doesn't remember the seizure and can usually resume full activity immediately.

Myoclonic seizures are sudden and consist of brief muscle contractions that may occur singly or repeatedly. Myoclonic seizures may involve the whole body in a massive jerk or spasm or may affect only individual limbs or muscle groups. If the myoclonic seizure involves the arms, it may cause the person to spill what he is holding. If the seizure involves the legs or body, the person may fall.

Tonic seizures are characterized by generalized muscle stiffening that lasts for about 1 to 10 seconds. This type of seizure is usually associated with many motor-related problems. The patient typically manifests an increased pulse, brief cessation of breathing, flushed face, bluish skin discoloration, and drooling. Fortunately, this seizure occurs mostly at night when the person is asleep. Since tonic seizures are quite sudden, if the seizure happens during the day the patient may fall violently and injure him or herself. This type of seizure is rare and usually occurs only in severe forms of epilepsy.

Atonic seizures produce a sudden loss of muscle tone, which, if brief, may only involve the patient's head dropping forward (head nods).

Appendix I: Complex Partial Seizures

A lengthier episode may cause a sudden collapse (drop attack). Drop attacks, also known as astatic seizures (Lipinski 1977), cause the patient to collapse but not lose consciousness. Patients recover completely within just a few minutes. Such attacks tend to occur late in the course of the patient's epilepsy, with average intervals noted of 11 years (Lipinski 1977), 12 years (Pazzaglia et al 1985), and 24 years (Gambardella et al. 1994).

Partial Seizures

In the United States, partial seizures are the most common type of seizures that occur after the first year of an individual's life. Internationally, there is insufficient data to compare the incidence to that in the United States; however, the incidence of epilepsy and the proportion of partial epilepsy are generally believed to be higher in developing countries because of the higher rates of infection and overall lower standards of health. In contrast to general seizures, partial seizures are focused in a limited area of the brain or only include one cerebral hemisphere. Partial seizures are categorized as simple partial seizures and complex partial seizures.

Simple partial seizures usually generate from one of the temporal lobes, and there is usually no impairment of consciousness. Although the patient's ability to respond may be preserved, motor manifestations or anxiety relating to the seizure symptoms may prevent a person experiencing a simple partial seizure from responding appropriately. The anatomical pathways involved in simple partial seizure determine the clinical symptoms. Simple partial seizures may be characterized by motor, sensory, psychic, or autonomic symptoms. Unlike other types of seizures, simple partial seizures may result in certain complex and interesting symptoms, such as déjà vu. This suggests that these types of seizures may have a more diffused rather than discrete localization.

In contrast, complex partial seizures occur when epileptic activity spreads to both temporal lobes. They often occur after a simple partial seizure of temporal lobe origin. Complex partial seizures do not involve convulsions, but consciousness is impaired. The patient will no longer respond to questions after the seizure starts. Complex partial seizures often begin with the person conveying a blank look or stare and may progress to chewing or uncoordinated activity. The patient may appear unaware of his or her surroundings and seem dazed.

Some patients perform meaningless behaviors that appear random and clumsy (automatisms). They may pick at their clothes or try to take them off, walk about, pick up things, or mumble. They may appear afraid and try to run or struggle with those who try to help. Complex partial seizures usually last for 2 to 4 minutes and may be followed by a state of confusion that lasts even longer. Once the pattern of the seizures is established in a given patient, it will usually be repeated with each subsequent seizure. Individuals with idiopathic, complex partial epilepsy may have a higher survival rate than those with symptomatic epilepsy and simple partial seizures.

AURAS

As discussed earlier, the term "aura" refers to the symptom or series of symptoms that occur prior to the onset of a seizure. The auras of complex partial seizures are particularly fascinating and often differ substantially from the auras of the other types of seizures. Although auras do not accompany all types of seizures, most patients with complex partial seizures report experiencing an aura before the seizure begins.

The most common type of aura is an epigastric sensation. This type of aura is typically associated with what Gowers calls "a nasty disagreeable smell." This symptom appears to be so distinctly unpleasant that in the late nineteenth century complex partial seizures were sometimes referred to as "uncinate fits," with reference to the olfactory center in the uncus. Other gustatory symptoms could also include an unpleasant and foul taste. Rarely, patients also report pleasant experiences, such as a sweet taste or scent.

Appendix I: Complex Partial Seizures

Somewhat less common auras are those known as illusions of familiarity (déjà vu or jamais vu) and affective symptoms (fear, anxiety, depression, vertigo, and nausea). During déjà vu, patients experience a sense of familiarity with the environment that they know is at variance with the facts. In déjà vu, patients—although clearly aware that they are, in fact, in a new and unfamiliar situation—feel that they have been there before or perhaps dreamt it before. In jamais vu, the opposite occurs. Patients, although clearly aware that they are in a customary and well-known situation, feel strongly that they have never been there before and that all is new or strange (Moore 1997). Uncommon auras include micropsia, hyperacusis, or hypoacusis, a sensation of hot or cold, palpitations, an urge to urinate, pain, and thirst.

Epileptic discharges in the middle and inferior temporal gyri can result in complex hallucinations or confusional episodes or may cause an abnormal attribution of emotional significance to otherwise neutral thoughts and external stimuli. Hallucinations become increasingly complex as the disturbance expands from primary to more complex association areas. A variety of emotional reactions can occur during the course of a temporal lobe seizure. Fear is the most frequently reported emotion during a seizure, but other reported emotions include anxiety, pleasure, displeasure, depersonalization, depression, familiarity, and unfamiliarity (Clark 1999). Complex hallucinations can cause patients to lose contact with reality and develop additional problems in their lives.

Visual hallucinations may vary in complexity from simple bright spots or geometric forms to detailed, almost cinematic, scenes. Auditory hallucinations also vary widely. They can include simple sounds, such as bells or mechanical noises, or highly complex sounds, such as instrumental music, songs, or voices.

> Auras may also appear in dreams. In cases in which the patient has long experienced auras and complex partial seizures during waking hours, the ictal nature of the dream content may be

fairly clear. However, in cases in which the epilepsy presents first only with isolated auras, and these auras appear only in dreams, the ictal nature of the repetitive dreams may be quite obscure and remain obscure until more obvious seizure activity occurs. (Moore 1997)

Epilepsy and Personality Change

The idea of personality change in people with epilepsy has been discussed for centuries. Even the ancient Greek physicians wrote descriptions about people with this condition. But because epilepsy is so pervasive and crosses so many cultural and geographical boundaries, it is difficult to develop a specific set of characteristics that are common to all epileptic patients. This is in sharp contrast to schizophrenia, which causes its victims to display a virtually universal pattern of symptoms and pathology. People with epilepsy have a variety of symptoms and different personality characteristics. There are, however, enough common characteristics among epileptics that researchers have been able to put together a fairly comprehensive picture of what is known as interictal personality disorder.

It should be noted that the current definition of interictal personality disorder is very different from the condition originally described by researchers in the nineteenth century, who put a much greater emphasis on a patient's affectivity. During the second half of the twentieth century, a new concept for defining the disorder was developed, particularly regarding complex partial seizures.

Viscosity and Hypergraphia

The writings of researcher Norman Geschwind have caused a great deal of debate and research in this area. According to Geschwind, people with an epileptic personality tend to have several common personality traits. These include viscosity with circumstantial speech and exaggerated and unnecessary preoccupation with religious and philosophical interests.

Appendix I: Complex Partial Seizures

The word "viscosity" typically relates to stickiness or adhesiveness. In 1982, two groups of researchers, Bear et al. and Rao et al., defined viscosity, with relation to the human psyche, as "a stickiness of thought processes but also . . . enhanced interpersonal adhesiveness." Viscosity causes the epileptic patient to talk repetitively and circumstantially, usually sticking to restricted topics. This "stickiness of thought process" presumably also accounts for the hypergraphia (a driving compulsion to write) that is often seen in these patients.

Geschwind provided an extensive description of this phenomenon in his research (Herman et al. 1988). People afflicted with hypergraphia compose writings that exceed social, occupational or educational requirements. The condition seems to stem from a pressing need in patients to express themselves and communicate their "sticky" ideas. These patients also tend to believe that their particular thoughts and ideas are unique and, therefore, must be written down.

In 1981, researches Sachdef and Waxman suggested that hypergraphia was more common in people with temporal lobe epilepsy than in those with other types of epilepsy. In 1993, Okamura et al. confirmed this finding, identifying temporal lobe epilepsy in 14 of 15 hypergraphic patients (93 percent) and finding temporal lobe involvement in only 19 of 32 of non-hypergraphic patients 59 percent (Moore 1997).

Religiosity and Sexuality

In the nineteenth century, Mosley reported that another feature often found in the epileptic patient was an exaggerated development of the religious sentiment (religiosity). In 1981, Kraepelin noted, "The religious content of the patients thought is another striking symptom, many patients spending a large part of their time in reading the Bible or praying aloud."

There also seems to be a correlation between complex partial seizures and sexuality. There are two sets of data available on this topic. In one series, researchers found hyposexuality, or a lack of sex drive, to be a prevailing problem in people with temporal lobe epilepsy. According to the researchers, the problem most commonly occurs when the seizures begin before the age of 12, when the patient's sexuality is still undeveloped. In a review of the sexual adjustment of 100 patients with medically intractable temporal lobe epilepsy, Taylor (1969) noted that the most common abnormality was low sexual drive but not failure of erection and ejaculation. Bloomer's global study in 1970 found hyposexuality in 58 percent of his 50 patients with intractable temporal lobe epilepsy.

In cases in which the patient's sexuality has developed and the onset of the disorder occurs after age 12, hypersexuality (excessive sexual activity) and sexual deviations are more prevalent. In 1991, Demorey et al. compared 127 female epileptic patients who had some form of sexual disorder with a match group of female epileptic patients with normal sexuality. The researchers discovered an increased prevalence of temporal lobe foci in the group with psychosexual disorders as compared to the sexually normal group.

Taking a somewhat different approach, Shukla et al. (1979) compared a group of 44 patients with temporal lobe foci to a group of 47 patients who had generalized discharge and found a greater degree of hyposexuality for men and women in the temporal lobe group as compared to the primary generalized group. The male test subjects showed a global loss of interest in sex, did not have erections, never had dreams or fantasies of a sexual nature, and had abandoned sexual intercourse altogether. The female test subjects, the authors noted, took part in sexual relations only after repeated requests from their husbands. When these females did consent, they remained totally passive and did not reach orgasm.

Taylor and Shukla et al. noted that the age of onset of epilepsy relative to the time of puberty had a significant impact on the patient's libido. There tended to be a loss of libido in patients with post-pubertal onset, whereas libido tended not to develop at all in patients with whom the epilepsy began before puberty. However, Shukla noted that regardless of the point at which libido was undeveloped or diminished, hyposexual patients had "no concern over the absent or diminished sexual functioning and none of them complained of it spontaneously."

In epileptic patients with hyposexuality, treatment with unilateral temporal lobotomy may lead to an increase in the person's sexuality. In 1967, Bloomer and Walker confirmed this finding in a study of 21 patients. Three years later, Bloomer expanded the study to 50 epileptic patients, 29 of which were found to be hyposexual preoperatively. Eight patients showed improved sexuality after the operation. Interestingly, improved sexuality was most likely to occur in those who experienced a substantial drop in seizure frequency post-operatively. Hyposexual patients who had minimal or no improvement in seizure frequency tended to remain hyposexual. On follow up, 8 patients who reported improved sexuality after surgery went on to develop hypersexuality that, in one case, was quite extreme (Moore 1997).

AGGRESSION

In 1981, researcher Emil Kraepelin noted that although there were a few patients who for years always displayed a placid disposition, most epileptic patients were easily angered and became threatening, quarrelsome, violent, and dangerous (Kraepelin 1981). The high prevalence of aggression among Kraepelin's patients may be explained, in part, by the fact that his practice was primarily limited to hospitalized patients.

In a similar vein, in 1965 Serafetinids assessed a highly select group of 100 patients with intractable temporal lobe seizures (most of whom were referred by psychiatric sources) and found overt physical aggressiveness in 36 percent of the patients. However, it is likely that the actual prevalence of aggressiveness among epileptic patients is much lower. Furthermore, lacking community-based studies, it is not even possible to say whether intractable aggressiveness is indeed more likely in epileptic patients than in a control group.

Given that some epileptics are clearly somewhat aggressive, it is worthwhile to consider some of the risk factors for aggression that occurred in this group of patients. Serafetinids thought that most of the aggressive patients had an early onset of epilepsy, but in his research he provided no statistical workup. He also thought that aggressiveness was more likely to occur in those patients with left dominant temporal lobe focus. Devinsky et al, utilizing the Buss-Durkee Hostility Inventory, subsequently noted that patients with a left temporal lobe focus scored higher on a suspicion scale than patients with right or bilateral temporal lobe focus. The left-lobe group appeared to harbor more resentment and hostility toward others than their calmer right-lobe counterparts.

In an attempt to construct a scale that would adequately express the nuances of interictal personality disorder, Bear and Fedio (1977) reviewed the literature on the disorder and came up with 18 traits that are characteristic of the syndrome. The researchers then used these 18 traits to construct a specific rating scale. Using this scale, they compared three groups: (1) patients with unilateral epileptic foci, (2) normal subjects, and (3) patients with neuromuscular disorders (Moore 1997).

PROPOSED INTERICTAL TRAITS

Trait	Clinical observations	Sample patient statements
Emotionality	Deepening of all emotions; sustained intense affect	My emotions have been so powerful that they have caused trouble.
Elation; euphoria	Grandiosity; exhilarated mood; diagnosis of manic-depressive disease	I have had periods when I feel so full of pep that sleep did not seem necessary for several days.

Appendix I: Complex Partial Seizures

Sadness	Discouragement; tearfulness; self-depreciation; diagnosis of depression; suicide	I have often felt so bad that I was close to ending my life.
Anger	Increased temper; Irritability	Little things make me angrier than they used to.
Aggression	Overt hostility; rage attacks; violent crime; murder	I have a tendency to break things or hurt people when I get angry.
Altered sexual interest	Loss of libido; hyposexualism; fetishism; transvestism; exhibitionism; hypersexual episodes	Things that never sexually attracted me before have become appealing.
Guilt	Tendency for self-scrutiny and self-recrimination	Much of the time I feel as if I have done something wrong or harmful.
Hypermoralism	Attention to rules with inability to distinguish significant from minor infraction; desire to punish offenders	I would go out of my way to make sure the law is followed.
Obsessionalism	Ritualism; orderliness; compulsive attention to detail	I have a habit of counting things or memorizing numbers.

Circumstantiality	Loquacious; pedantic; overly detailed; peripheral	People sometimes tell me that I have trouble getting to the point because of all the details
Viscosity	Stickiness; tendency for repetition	Sometimes I keep at a thing so long that others may lose their patience with me.
Sense of personal destiny	Events given highly charged; personalized significance; ascribed to many features of patient's life	I think I have a special mission in life.
Hypergraphia	Keeping extensive diaries; de-tailed notes; writing auto-biography or novel	I write down or copy many things.
Religiosity	Holding deep religious beliefs; often idiosyncratic; multiple conversions; mystical states	I have had some very unusual religious experiences.
Philosophical interest	Nascent metaphysic or moral speculations; cosmologic theories	I have spent a lot of time thinking about the origins of the world and life.
Dependency; passivity	Cosmic helplessness; "at hands of fate;" protestations of others.	I feel like a pawn in the hands of others.

Appendix I: Complex Partial Seizures

Humorlessness; sobriety	Over generalized ponderous concern; humor lacking or idiosyncratic	People should think about the point of many jokes more carefully instead of just laughing at them.
Paranoia	Suspicious; over interpretive of motives and events; diagnosis of paranoid schizophrenia	People tend to take advantage of me.

(Table taken from Moore 1997, 182)

Behavioral Changes and The Brain

Even with all this current knowledge regarding the brain, behavior, and complex partial seizures, there is some related material regarding temporal lobes and schizophrenia that can shed light on the causes of the behavioral changes that are brought on by complex partial seizures. It is now accepted that dysfunction of the dorsolateral region of the temporal lobe may be associated with several psychopathological states. Temporal lobe lesions due to a variety of neurological insults (harm) can lead a patient to present signs and symptoms that are more consistent with a psychiatric diagnosis than with a traditional neurological one (Clark 1999). Although schizophrenia and complex partial seizures are two entirely different conditions, there is an inherent correlation between the two diseases. It appears that, at least partially, these two conditions are heavily correlated due to their involvement with the temporal lobes.

During the last 50 years, there has been an abundance of research produced that indicates there is a loss of volume in the brains of schizophrenics. A reduction in volume of the superior temporal gyros in schizophrenia was suspected for some time (Southard 1910), but only confirmed recently (Barta et al. 1990). The effect appears to be specific to the dominant cortex, especially in males (Reite et al. 1997). In addition, there is a strong correlation between the increase of thought disorder and volume reduction in the left posterosuperior temporal gyros (McCarley et al. 1993a). By comparison, there is a close association between auditory hallucinations and volume reduction in the more anterior regions of the superior temporal gyros (Barta et al. 1990). These findings are consistent with the findings that there is greater impairment in auditory processing than in visual processing in schizophrenia (Clark 1999).

Apparently, one of the main functions of the temporal lobes is to regulate senses, instincts, and emotions. The tissue of these lobes consists of large neurons, which bring the information to the temporal lobes and small neurons, which have an inhibitory effect by triggering a series of interneurons that are connected to the long ones. Although many pieces of information regarding each sense or emotion comes to this part of the brain, the small neurons modulate and control this information so that just enough of it is brought to the person's attention to enable him or her to function and focus on the task at hand. However, due to the limited number of inhibitory neurons in schizophrenic patients, the person cannot control these pieces of information and develops serious disturbances of the senses that manifest in the form of hallucinations, delusions, inappropriate behavior, and inability to distinguish between reality and unreality.

There is also an abundance of research that suggests a similar mechanism is responsible for the problems associated with temporal lobe epilepsy (Denslow et al. 2001). Apparently, the electrical stimulation caused by the seizure does the same thing to the brain that volume loss does in schizophrenics. Therefore, the person manifests similar symptoms of hallucination and improper control of emotions. When the areas in the brain related to control of sexuality and aggression are not controlled, problems of hyposexuality or hypersexuality, extremes of aggression, poor initiation, and the other symptoms mentioned above result. In addition, there is some evidence that the left temporal lobe has some impact on human religiosity—distortion of a person's religiosity both among schizophrenics and people suffering from complex partial seizure can be observed.

The episodes of seizures are a small portion of an epileptic's life, so the impact on a person's psyche and the symptoms are not as intense for an epileptic as a schizophrenic. Consequently, the devastation caused to the brain is more tolerable for epileptics, and their ability to function in society is much better than for schizophrenics. However, once these experiences are prolonged, people afflicted with this disease reflect a personality style that is religious and aggressive and have an unusual sex life and sense of mission. In other words, the temporal lobe in its dysfunction can be observed, which is then called interictal personality.

The symptoms of aura, seizure, and postictal symptoms could all be explained within the context of anatomy and functions of the temporal lobe (Denslow et al 2001, 86:2231–2245). It should also be noted that there are many new theories regarding the causes and effects of epilepsy However, the purpose this book is not to answer all of these questions but to provide some general knowledge regarding the seizure disorder in order to understand this discussion. Without doubt, future advances in medicine will be able to shed better light on this devastating condition.

APPENDIX II

HISTORICAL & RELIGIOUS FIGURES SUGGESTED IN THE MEDICAL LITERATURE TO HAVE HAD EPILEPSY

Person	Description of Spells	Frequency	Likelihood of Epilepsy	Differential Diagnosis [a]	Religious Aspects
Margery Kempe (ca. 1373–1438)	A cry, falling with convulsive movements, turning blue, nausea, Psychotic behavior	Recurrent	+	Epilepsy Hysteria postpartum psychosis Migraine	14th-century Christian mystic and autobiographer
Joan of Arc (1412–1431)	I heard this Voice [of an angel] . . . accompanied also by a . . . great light . . . there is never a day when I do not hear this Voice; and I have much need of it."	At least daily by the time of her execution in 1431	+	ecstatic partial seizure and musciogenic epilepsy Intracranial tuberculoma	Extraordinary, deeply held, idiosyncratic religious beliefs motivating martial prowess in the defense of Orléans
St. Catherine of Genoa (1447–1510)	Extreme sense of heat or cold, whole-body tremor, transient aphasia, automatisms, sense of passivity, hyperesthesia, regression to childhood, dissociation, sleepwalking, transient weakness, transient suggestibility, inability to open eyes	Unknown	+	Complex partial seizure Hysteria	Christian mystic

Appendix II: Historical & religious figures suggested in the medical literature to have had epilepsy

St. Teresa of Ávila (1515–1582)	Visions, chronic headaches, transient LOC, tongue-biting	1 major LOC spell; frequent headaches	++	Complex partial seizure Hysteria	Catholic saint
St. Catherine dei Ricci (1522–1590)	LOC, visual hallucinations, mystical states	Every Thursday at noon with recovery by Friday at 4:00 P.M.	+	Complex partial seizure	Catholic saint
Emanuel Swedenborg (1688–1772)	Acute psychosis, foaming at the mouth, olfactory, gustatory, and somatic hallucinations, ecstatic aura, falling LOC, convulsions, hallucinations, postictal trance states	Recurrent	++	Complex partial seizure Mania Schizophrenia	Founder of the New Jerusalem Church

Ann Lee (1736–1784)	Visual, auditory hallucinations	From childhood until at least 1774	+	Epilepsy	Founder of the Shaker movement
Joseph Smith (1805–1844)	Speech arrest, fear, "pillar of light," hearing voices, "When I came to... I found myself lying on my back looking up at heaven	One clear conversion event (1820)	+	Complex partial seizure	Founder of Mormonism
Fyodor Mikhailovitch Dostoyevsky (1821–1881)	Sense of bliss, then a cry, a fall, generalized tonic-clonic seizure with frothing at the mouth and injuries Postictal intense depression and guilt, lasting several days	Every few days to every few months	+++	Complex partial seizure with generalization Primary generalized seizures Hysteria	Influential Russian novelist Ecstatic auras: "I have really touched God. He came into me myself; yes, God exists, I cried, and I don't remember anything else." Interictal religiosity increasing with age.

Appendix II: Historical & Religious Figures Suggested in the Medical Literature to Have Had Epilepsy

Hieronymus Jaegen (1841–1919)	Mystical experiences, visual hallucinations, headaches	Unknown	+	Complex partial seizure Migraine	German mystic
Dr. Z (Arthur Thomas Myers; 1851–1894)	Pallor, vacant look, preservation of "yes" to any remark, tongue smacking, *déjà vu*, right-sided motor signs, postictal passivity	Multiple episodes 1871–1894	+++	Complex partial seizures Left temporal lobe lesion on autopsy	Late-life interest in afterlife, reincarnation; prominent in the Society for Psychical Research
Vincent Van Gogh (1853–1890)	Sense of vertigo, tinnitus, hyperacusis, xanthopsia, restlessness, delirium Digitalis intoxication	About 1 dozen spells between the ages of 35 and 37	+	Complex partial seizure with postictal psychosis Ménière's disease Meningoencephalitis luetica Schizophrenia	Renowned painter Hyperreligiosity
St. Thérèse of Lisieux (1873–1897)	Violent trembling, visual hallucinations, wounding by a "shaft of fire," mystical conversions	Several spells after age 9	++	Complex partial seizure	Catholic saint

BIBLIOGRAPHY

African Commission on Human and People's Rights. 2004. *Statement on the Current Human Rights Situation in Darfur, Sudan, Delivered on 23 May 2004.* http://www.antislavery.org/archive/submission/Africacommission2004-Darfur.htm.

Al-Tabari, M. 1990. *Tarikh Tabari* (Persian), vol. 3–4, trans. by A. Paiandeh. Tehran, Iran: Sherkat Entesharat Asatir.

Al-Bukhari M. 1988. *The Translation of the Meanings of Sahih* (Arabic and English), vol. 1–9. Chicago, IL: Kazi Publications.

Adams, Francis, ed. 1856. *The Extant Works of Aretaeus, the Cappadocian.* London, U.K.: Wertheimer and Company.

Armstrong, Karen. 1992. *Muhammad: A Biography of the Prophet.* New York: HarperCollins.

Blumer, D. 1999. "Evidence Supporting the Temporal Lobe Epilepsy Personality Syndrome." *Neurology,* 53(5 Suppl. 2):s9–12.

Boyce, M. 1995. *A History of Zoroastrianism* (Persian). Tehran, Iran: Publisher unknown.

Clark, David, Nashaat Boutros, and Mario Mendez. 2005. *The Brain and Behavior: An Introduction to Behavioral Neuroanatomy.* Cambridge University Press.

Dashti, A. 1994. *Twenty Three Years: A Study of the Prophetic Career of Mohammad* (English), trans. F.R.C. Bagley. Costa Mesa, CA: Mazda Publications.

Dashti, A. *Twenty Three Years* (Persian). Publisher and dates unknown.

Denslow, Maria, Tore Eid, Fu Du, Robert Schwartz, Eric W. Lothman, and Oswald Steward. 2001. "Disruption of Inhibition in Area CA1 of Hippocampus in a Rat Model of Temporal Lobe Epilepsy." *Journal of Neurophysiology,* 86(5):2231–2245.

Devinsky, O., and S. Najjar. 1999. "Evidence Against the Existence of a Temporal Lobe Personality Syndrome." *Neurology* 53(5 Suppl. 2): s12–s25.

Engel, J. 1996. "Introduction to Temporal Lobe Epilepsy." *Epilepsy Research* 26(1) (December):141–150.

Freeman, F. 1976. "A Differential Diagnosis of the Inspirational Spells of Muhammad, the Prophet of Islam." *Epilepsia* 17(4) (December):423–427.

Geschwind, N. 198. "Interictal Behavioral Changes in Epilepsy." *Epilepsia* 24 (Suppl. 1):S23–S30.

Goldziher, I. 1889 (1971 reprint). *Muslim Studies,* vol. 1–2, trans. by C.R. Barber and S.M. Stern. London, U.K.: George Allen and Unwin Ltd.

Ibn Ishaq, Sirat Rasul, A. Guillaume, trans. 1955. *The Life of Muhammad: A Translation of Ibn Ishaq's Sirat Rasul Allah.* London: Oxford University Press.

Heical. M. 1966. *The Life of Muhammad* (Persian translation), vol. 1–2. Tehran, Iran: Elmi Publishers (6th edition).

Hitti, Phillip. 1996. *The Arabs: A Short History.* Washington, D.C.: Regency Publishing.

Ibn Saad, M. 1990. *Al Tabaghat Al Cobra* (Arabic), vol. 1–2. Beirut, Lebanon: Dar Al Kotob Elmi.

Ireland, W. 1886 (1972 reprint). *The Blot upon the Brain: Studies in History and Psychology.* Freeport, NY: Books for Libraries Press.

Korkut, D. 2001. Life Alert: *The Medical Case of Mu*hammad. Enumclaw, WA: WinePress Publishing.

Ling, M. 1983. *Muhammad, His Life Based on Earliest So*urces. Rochester, VT: Inner Traditions International.

Lishman, W. 1997. *Organic Psychiatry: The Psychological Consequences of Cerebral Disorder* (3rd Ed.). London, U.K.: Blackwell Science.

Makarem Shirazi, M. Ayatollah. 1995. *Tafsir Nemouneh* (Persian), vol. 1–29. Tehran, Iran: Dar Al Kotob Al Islamieh.

Mostofi, H. 1988. *Tarikh Gozidh* (Persian) Tehran, Iran: Entesharat Amir Kabir.

Moore, D. 1997. *Partial Seizures and Interictal Disorders, the Neuropsychiatric Elements*. Boston, MA: Butterworth-Heinemann.

Noldeke, T. 1892 (1963 reprint). *Sketches from Eastern History*, trans. J.S. Black. Beirut, Lebanon: Khayats.

Read, D. 1981. "Solving Deductive-reasoning Problems After Unilateral Temporal Lobectomy." *Brain and Language*, 12:116–127.

Saver, J. 1997. "The Neural Substrates of Religious Experience." *Journal of Neuropsychiatry* 9(3) (Summer):498.

Seguy, M. R. 1977. *Miraj Nameh* (Turkish). Paris, France: George Braziller.

Shakir. M., trans. 1990. *The Quran* (English translation). Chicago, IL: Kazi Publications.

Sobhani, J. 1994. *Forough e Abaddiat: Comprehensive Analysis of the Prophet's Life* (Persian). Tehran, Iran: Danesh Islami.

Suhaili, A.R. 1977. *Al sirat Al Nabavia* (Arabic) Pakistan

Turner. A. 1993. *The History of Hell*. New York: Harvest Books.

Valliant, G. 1986. *Empirical Studies of Ego Mechanisms of Defense. Washington, D.C.:* American Psychiatric Press.

Waghedy .M. 1986. *Al Moghazi* (Persian), Translated by Mahdavi Damghani, M. vol. 1–3. Tehran, Iran: Markaz Nashr Daneshgahi

Waxman, S. 1975. "The Interictal Behavior Syndrome in Temporal Lobe Epilepsy." *Archives of General Psychiatry* 32(12) (December):1580–1586.

Wintle, J. 2003. *The Rough Guide History of Islam*. London, U.K.: Rough Guide Publishers.

Yusuf Ali, A. 1987. *The Holy Quran: Text, Translation and Commentary*. Elmhurst, NY: Tahrike Tarsile Quran.

To order additional copies of this title call:
1-877-421-READ (7323)
or please visit our web site at
www.annotationbooks.com